Super Health Thru Organic Super Food

R. W. Bernard

This scarce antiquarian book is included in our special *Legacy Reprint Series*. In the interest of creating a more extensive selection of rare historical book reprints, we have chosen to reproduce this title even though it may possibly have occasional imperfections such as missing and blurred pages, missing text, poor pictures, markings, dark backgrounds and other reproduction issues beyond our control. Because this work is culturally important, we have made it available as a part of our commitment to protecting, preserving and promoting the world's literature. Thank you for your understanding.

DEDICATION

This book is dedicated to two great humanitarians, Anton H. Jensen and Dr. M. A. Brandon, who have done so much to pioneer the new Organic Food Movement which is now sweeping across the country, as more and more people, as the result of the great work of Jensen and Brandon in publishing and spreading my findings and writings on food reform, are realizing the grave menace to their health that lies hidden in foods grown with chemical fertilizers and sprays, and the great importance of using only organically grown foods, which are free from these poisons. The author also gratefully pays homage to America's greatest living agricultural reformer, J. I. Rodale, editor of "Organic Gardening and Farming" and "Prevention", for the valuable work that he has done to initiate and spread the Organic Movement in America.

FOREWORD

The present book is the sequel of the book "How to Eat Safely In A Poisoned World, published by the writer's friend and colleague, Anton H. Jensen, on the basis of a manuscript by this name which the writer furnished Mr. Jensen, with permission to edit and publish it under his own name. On the last page of this book appeared an announcement of its sequel, this present work, which Mr. Jensen asked the writer to write and which he would print, as he did the other book, in his print shop in Lincoln, Nebraska. (Jensen was a printer by profession.)

The book "How to Eat Safely In A Poisoned World" dealth largely with the men poisoning of our foods by arsenic and lead insecticides and the importance of unsprayed, organically grown foods. Since this book was written, the older arsenical sprays have been largely replaced by the new more powerful DDT derivatives, which it is the purpose of the following pages to discuss. Also, the new science of organic dietetics, which was in its infancy when the first book was published, has made considerable headway since then, and there are many new developments in organic foods and organic nutrition which will be presented in the following pages.

Since he wrote the "Jensen" book, the writer has written a number of other works on food poisoning by sprays and the importance of organic foods, including "Are The New Super Sprays Endangering Your Health?", dealing with DDT, chlordane and other newly developed super-powerful insecticides, "Are You Being Poisoned By the Foods You Eat?", "Organic Foods For Health", "Health Through Scientific Nutrition" (How to Go an Organic Diet for Health Regeneration), a study course on "The Organic Way to Health" and "Are Chemicals in Drinking Water Menacing your Health?", also "Revolt Against Chemicals" and "The Organic Revolution in Nutrition".

The purpose of the above works is to show how it is possible to keep in good health under the abnormal conditions of modern civilization, whose food and water supply are poisoned by chemicals in the form of chemical fertilizers, sprays, preservatives, additives, chlorine, fluorine and other chemicals added to drinking water, etc. After pointing out the danger lurking in ordinary foods and water, the writer has pointed out the benefits to health of organically grown foods and glass-distilled water (prepared at home in a glass distillator, rather than using commerical distilled water made in a metallic apparatus and which is, for this reason, not 100% pure).

The fundamental idea on which this book is based is that if one hopes to achieve the highest degree of health, it is necessary to live on strictly organic diet. Such a diet differs radically from what modern nutritionists consider an "optimal" diet for health, which, in their opinion, means a diet rich in all nutritional essentials, such as amine acids, vitamins, minerals, etc. The new conception in nutrition which this book presents is that health depends on much more than this. A diet might supply large amounts of all nutritional essentials - the whole family of amino acids, the whole alphabet of vitamins, the whole series of minerals, etc. - and still fail miserably to support good health; and, instead, might bring on disease. For, according to the viewpoint here maintained, health fundamentally depends on <u>the manner in which foods were grown</u> - on the soil on which they were raised, the kind of fertilizers used in their production, the presence or absence of insecticide residues in them, etc. Only foods grown in a natural manner, without the use of chemicals or sprays, according to the new nutritional viewpoint which this book upholds, are capable of supporting good health - no matter how high they may be in vitamins, minerals, complete proteins and other nutrients revealed by chemical analysis. A high mineral content, for example, does not necessarily mean that the food is capable of supplying a correspondingly large percentage of <u>available</u> minerals, since, if foods are grown with chemical fertilizers, a certain part of their mineral content will be in inorganic form, in the form of chemical fertilizer residues, which the body cannot use. Only when foods are grown organically, without chemicals, are all their minerals in organic combination, and therefore available for bodily use. It is a fact that chemical fertilizers, being more readily soluble than the natural colloidal minerals of the soil, will tend to be more quickly appropriated by the roots of plants, and so will replace soil minerals in the plant's metabolism. And while plants grown with chemicals might show on analysis a high mineral content, perhaps higher than those grown naturally, we should bear in mind that these minerals are qualitatively different from the natural organically combined minerals of normal plant tissues, in which, under such conditions, it may be markedly deficient, due to their replacement by inorganic minerals derived from chemical fertilizer residues.

It is therefore clear that it is not merely the quantitative chemical analysis of foods that is important, but certain hitherto neglected qualitative factors must be considered. Just as synthetic vitamins manufactured in the chemical laboratory differ from the natural vitamins of organic foods, so the minerals, and the vitamins into which they are elaborated, of plants grown with chemicals differ from those present in foods grown naturally. Plants certainly were never intended by nature to feed on chemicals, but on soil mineral colloids derived from decomposed rock material; and it is therefore clear that chemical fertilizer residues in foods must act as foreign impurities, or toxins, which, by disturbing normal mineral metabolism, create mineral and vitamin deficiency in plants and in animals and humans that feed on chemically fertilized produce. By interfering with the normal biochemical equilibrium of living cells, such chemical fertilizer residues, taken up from the soil by plants and communicated by them to animals and human beings, in the opinion of Keens in England, Holder in Canada and Rodale in America, constitute an important etiological factor contributing to the modern increase of cancer in all countries where chemical fertilizers are in common use.

More and more progressive nutritionists are today in agreement that only foods grown without chemical fertilizers or poisonous sprays are capable of supporting good health. And since such foods are not generally available in most so-called civilized countries, where mass production by chemical methods of agriculture is the rule, it is clear that if good health depends on naturally grown foods, it cannot be found among those who live on chemicalized foods, which fact is proven by the widespread diseases that today plague nations which feed on the products of chemical agriculture. It is necessary to look outside of civilization and far away from it, in lands where life and agriculture are primitive and natural, and where the practices of chemical fertilization and spraying are unknown, to find genuinely healthy specimens of the human species.

For nine years, a world-famous nutritional scientist, Dr. Robert McCarrison, as a British medical officer, lived among such a race in the far-off Himalayas, during which time he conducted a careful study of their diet and agricultural practices in relation to their health. These people, known as the Hunzas, he found to be entirely disease-free. They were entirely exempt from all of the common diseases that afflict civilized races, such as appendicitis, heart and kidney ailments, cancer, etc. What was the reason for their unusual immunity to the diseases from which other races suffer was the object of his special research.

Dr. McCarrison found the solution of this problem in their diet; and he also found that it was not only the type of foods the Hunzas ate that accounted for their remarkable health, but the manner in which they cultivated the soil on which they grew their foods. As for their diet, except for the rare or occasional use of goat meat, it was practically vegetarian. No cow's meat, no cow's milk or dairy products, no eggs, no fish, no refined sugar or cereals and no canned foods were used. Goat milk was the only milk used; and this was taken in soured form. The base of their diet consisted of apricots, millet, chick peas, buckwheat, vegetables, and some potatoes, a food which was introduced among them comparatively recently.

But mere selection of foods did not explain the extraordinary health and vigor of these long-lived, disease-free people, since many vegetarians in this country live on a similar diet, yet are far from specimens of health. Nor could the pure mountain air they breathed account for the superior health which the Hunzas enjoyed, since neighboring races, whose manner of living was different from their's, were poor examples of health and suffered from many diseases. The secret of the Super-Health of the Hunzas Dr. McCarrison discovered in their diet of Organic Super Foods grown on Super Soil. For the soil that produced the foods that they consumed was not ordinary soil. Not only was it free from chemical poisons, derived from fertilizers and sprays, which contaminate the soil on which most American foods have been grown, but it was very rich in the two prime essentials of soil fertility - humus, derived from decayed organic matter, and natural mineral colloids, derived from decomposed rocks. The latter were communicated to the soil by irrigation water coming from the mountains above, carrying silt worn away from decomposed rocks by the grinding action of glaciers. The conscientious Hunza organic gardener also returned to the soil the organic matter removed by growing crops, thus completing the "wheel of health", described by an English physician Wrench, in his book on the Hunzas bearing this title. From a Super Soil the Hunzas derived Super Foods; and on a diet of Organic Super Foods they acquired a state of Super Health. Such is the lesson and message of the Hunzas, which constitutes the keynote of this book, a message first announced to the scientific world by McCarrison, later re-echoed by his countryman Wrench; and finally brought to the American people by Rodale, in his book "The Healthy Hunzas".

In writing this book, the author's purpose is to show that what the Hunzas have done, we, too, can do; and we can likewise enjoy Super Health if we live on a diet of Organic Super Foods. In the following pages the writer wishes to outline the basic principle of a new science of nutrition based on this new point of view; and to show how it is possible to transfer the general state of so-called "health" (really a condition of continual aches, pains and discomforts, not to mention periodic colds, headaches, periods of illness, etc., and universal tooth decay - in short, a condition generally defined as one not sick enough to require being confined to bed) into one of SUPER HEALTH, as enjoyed by the Hunzas, a very unusual physiological state, involving complete immunity to diseases of all kinds, something almost never observed among so-called civilized people who live on commercially produced foods, raised by the use of chemical fertilizers and sprays.

The writer hopes to follow this book with a sequel, to which the last chapter, entitled "Super Health From Super Soil", is devoted. This new book will deal with the methods of growing Organic Super Foods by an entirely new innovation in agricultural practice, which is not only different from conventional methods of chemical fertilization and spraying, but is far in advance of the organicultural method based on the use of composts derived from animal and vegetable humus, earthworms, etc. The writer maintains that only by the growing of Super Foods on a Super Soil which has been prepared and cultivated by the new method can a Super Race arise, a race free from diseases of all kinds, enjoying a remarkable longevity and achieving a degree of brain development hitherto unknown. For since it is a biological truism that the human being is a chemical derivative of the foods consumed, and since foods are derived from the soil, by creating a new Super Soil, it should be possible to create a new Super Man. All readers of this book who are interested in the new book and who wish to hasten their receiving it are requested to write to the publisher and send in their advance unpaid order. This will do much to encourage the publisher to proceed all the more rapidly with publication of the forthcoming book, "Super Foods From Super Soil".

Chapter One

MORE AND MORE DEADLY SPRAYS TO POISON YOU FASTER

In years gone by arsenic and lead were considered to be the arch chemo-enemies of human health, present in sprayed vegetables and fruits. But as dangerous as arsenic and lead are, in comparison with the newly developed super-destructive insecticides, such as chlordane, they are what the first Hiroshima bomb was in comparison with the latest hydrogen bomb. This is an excellent comparison, for in either case, scientific "progress" has been in the direction of exterminating life - including human life - more effectively and efficiently. While bombs are intended primarily for annihilating human beings, and while insecticides are intended to kill insect pests, just as bombs can also kill insects, so insecticides can also kill human beings.

Starting with DDT, a whole series of increasingly more toxic insecticides have been developed in recent years, known as chlorinated hydrocarbons, most well known among which is chlordane, a highly toxic lethal agent, dangerous to insects and also human beings, whether taken in through the mouth, nose or skin. These new super-toxic insecticides were perfected in rapid succession, one more poisonous than the other. Since greater toxicity meant an economic saving to the grower, who had to use less of a more toxic spray than of a less toxic one, a death race went on among manufacturers of insecticides for the purpose of capturing the market by offering to growers the most highly toxic insecticide possible. As a result, new poisons were perfected and placed on the market which were ghastly in their destructiveness.

The DDT Spray Menace

The following excellent summary of the essential facts concerning DDT and its menace to modern life appeared in the February 1954 issue of Herald of Health, a publication of the drugless profession, in an article, "The Poisoning of Americans":

"We, naturopaths, have watched the growing list of poisons that have entered into our country's economy and have long realized that the day is not far distant when this continuous doping will lead to nationwide disaster. The only question seems to be - just how many Americans will survive this slow, cumulative bombardment of killing substances to be here when the final catastrophe arrives.

"During the Second World War, down in the Pacific, the medical brass hats with the army - working with the poison gas experts in the Chemical Warfare Department - brought into being an insecticide which was immediately named DDT because its long scientific title went close to thirty letters. This deadly concoction was very effective when sprinkled or sprayed about the army camps. It killed the flies and the mosquitoes, the crawly things and the moths, the birds and the smaller animals - in fact, it made the undergrowth of the jungle, which usually teems with small life, a barren sepulcher.

"After the war, the manufacturers of this potent killer dampened it down a trifle and added to it the poisons that have been gradually saturating the bodies of our people for a generation. And when this milder DDT went into action on the home front in the hands of the fruit grower, the gardener and orchardist, the same results followed as had occurred in the jungle - insects and smaller animals gave up the ghost in countless billions. In California alone, more than one-fourth of the honey bees died within three months and all living things fled before DDT's deadly mists. And this insidious poison defied all efforts of the housewife to cleanse it entirely from the skins of fruits and vegetables. Washington officials expressed themselves as not alarmed that this dangerous substance still clung to the food eaten by the majority of Americans. They said it was in such small amounts that it did no OBSERVABLE harm. No, because it did not KILL INSTANTLY it was considered SAFE by the chuckle-headed, dollar-crazed bunch that supposedly was protecting the health of all Americans.

"Now a New York City physician, by the name of W. Coda Martin, has come forward with some startling facts about food poisoning and DDT in particular. This metropolitan doctor examined the fatty tissues of 25 of his patients chosen at random, and he discovered that 23 had really sizeable amounts of DDT stored in their bodies. Now these patients live in the great city of New York - and they never had occasion to handle DDT in any manner. So the only conclusion that can be drawn is that this poison came to them on or in the food they ate. It indicates that all Americans - yes, folks in every city, town and village of this country who have to eat fruits and vegetables which have been sprayed with DDT to kill marauding insects and rusts - are now building up in the cells of their bodies huge stores of this poison that will shorten their lives materially. Yet most of these persons have been careful in their selection of food, have been sure that the vegetables and fruits they ate were thoroughly washed. It was good old Dr. Weyland J. Hayes, chief toxicologist of the United States Health Service, who observed calmly that despite all the washing of fruit and vegetables 'varying amounts of these poisonous residues remain, which are absorbed by the human body with food.' It was his profound opinion, however, that 'there is little proof of toxic effects of these substances in the human body and therefore the danger of chronic toxicity (poisoning) is negligible.' This was exactly opposite to the findings of Dr. Martin with his 23 patients.

"Dr. Martin, in his published report of this DDT poisoning went on to say: 'DDT is poisonous to man as well as insects and the fearful possibilities are shown in the statement of the Department of Agriculture that more than 250 million pounds of this potent poison are now being used by the fruit and vegetable raisers in the country.' And he added, ' it is well known scientifically that the chlorinated hydrocarbons - of which DDT is one - are cumulative in animal and human fats. This means that such poisons - including DDT - when taken into the human body do not pass through, but are piled up in the cells in ever-increasing amounts. '

"Dr. Martin is right. Most naturopaths have found evidence of this growing poison in many of their patients. And as the use of DDT and its kindred killers is increasing with each passing year, the damage to the liver and other eliminative organs is growing. Just figure out what will happen if this damage is not halted - just imagine the condition of millions upon millions of Americans at the end of say ten or fifteen years from now!

"Of course there is a remedy - a direct remedy - but it is so far out of <u>ordinary</u> procedure that it would be impossible to take advantage of it. If a man gives another a dose of arsenic or other poison, and the one who drinks it dies, we have a charge of murder involved. What difference is there when a farmer in an attempt to kill destroying insects loads his vegetables or his fruit with poisons which he passes on to you as the consumer, without making any effort to free his food of these dangerous substances? Isn't he just as guilty as the man who intentionally gives arsenic to another?

"So the remedy for these conditions is to pass laws that all produce sold in the marketplace MUST be totally free of poison or the producer of such produce will be prosecuted in the courts. That would end this poison-menace overnight!

"Fifty years ago, garden produce did not need poisons to protect it from insects and blights. The rich natural soil brought into being only robust, healthy plants which could protect themselves. Today, the farmer and gardener raises larger plants - <u>but not healthy ones.</u> These bloated individuals have to be protected in some manner or the insects would destroy them before they reached maturity.

"If the farmer will go back to natural fertilization, he will solve his insect problems, will raise better food and will not be slowly killing his customers. Natural fertilization is possible today and the quicker the son-of-the-soil realizes that the poisonous chemicals he now uses as fertilizer merely kills the fertility of his land - the sooner he will be on the road to save his farm instead of ruining it.

"Let us repeat again - to stop this poisoning, laws should be passed making a farmer, gardener or food processor criminally responsible if even a TRACE OF POISON is found on the product sold by such a farmer, gardener or food processor. That is a simple solution to a desperate situation that is becoming more vital with each passing day. And DDT - the latest comer in this field - should be the first to be kicked out."

In the winter of 1949, a sensational series of articles appeared in the New York Post entitled "DDT and You". The author, Albert Deutsch, cites the findings of Dr. Morton S. Biskind, New York physician and pharmacologist, concerning the health menace of DDT residues in vegetables, fruits, meat and milk, resulting from the spraying of crops and cows with this poison. Deutsch quotes Dr. Biskind's view that the increasing prevalence of virus "X" disease is caused by contamination of foods, especially milk, with DDT. This new nerve disease, he points out, was unknown before this new insecticide was first introduced. He calls attention to the alarming fact that millions of babies are being slowly poisoned by DDT present in the milk they drink, this poison being also present in butter, cheese and meat sold to the public. According to Deutsch, DDT is such a powerful nerve poison that even years after exposure to minute traces of it, the nervous system will show its after-effects. "DDT", he writes, "can be toxic to man in incredibly small amounts." DDT, which is sprayed on cows to protect them from insects, is absorbed through their skin or inhaled through their respiratory tract, and is thus communicated to meat and milk. Other ways in which cows take in this poison is from the spraying of their food, their barn, or the pasture on which they feed. The poison is stored in the fatty tissues; and, in the case of humans, damage to the liver or nervous system may not be apparent until ten to twenty years later. All dairy products produced from sprayed cows or in sprayed barns may be dangerous. This includes butter, ice cream, condensed milk, etc.

It was not long after Deutsch's series of articles appeared, revealing the wholesale poisoning of the American people by DDT, that the powerful financial clique behind its sale exerted sufficient pressure to gag him; and he has been silent ever since.

Dr. Martin's Studies on Widespread DDT Poisoning

Four years after Deutsch's sensational articles on DDT mass poisoning appeared in the <u>New York Post</u>, a United Press report appeared in the <u>New York World-Telegram</u> on Dept. 15, 1953, which awoke national interest. The article dealt with the researches of a New York physician, Dr. Coda Martin, on DDT poisoning, which he found to be an almost universal condition among the American people. Since DDT was employed on an ever-increasing scale since the time when Deutsch's articles appeared, with the result that 90% of the specimens of meat and milk picked at random in public markets recently showed the presence of DDT - as was found in the fatty tissues of a similar percentage of New Yorkers studied by Dr. Martin - it is clear that the situation is far more serious today than it was four years ago. We quote from the article on Dr. Martin's findings, referred to above:

"MD FEARS DDT IS POISONING NATION, FINDS TRACES IN 23 OF 25 HUMANS
By Delos Smith, United Press Science Editor

"A New York physician subjected samples of fatty tissues taken from 25 New Yorkers who had never handled DDT, except momentarily, to chemical analysis and found DDT in 23.

"This caused the physician, Dr. Coda Martin, to ask fellow practitioners last night - 'What will happen to the entire population in 10 to 15 years from now?'

"Addressing the New York chapter of the American Academy of Nutrition, Dr. Martin said his patients accumulated DDT in their bodies from DDT insecticides on or in the food they ate.

"<u>DDT Poisonous to Man</u>

"DDT is poisonous to man as well as to insects, he said, adding that the use of DDT and its chemical relatives in agriculture now totals well over 250,000,000 pounds a year and is increasing.

"He said that because the chlorinated hydrocarbons - of which DDT is one - 'are known to be accumulative in animal and human fats, it is essential that further studies be made of the chronic toxic effects on the human in order to protect the future health of the nation.'

"'Chronic poisoning (from chlorinated hydrocarbons) produces severe degenerative changes in the liver, the most severely damaged of the vital organs', he said. 'Although DDT produces serious morphological (structural) changes in virtually every organ of the body, its most disturbing effects are those of the nervous system.'

"Warns of Liver Damage

"Dr. Martin said laboratory analysis showed that the DDT level in the 23 out of 25 human fatty tissue samples examined ranged from one part per million to 11 parts per million.

"In response to an inquiry from this reporter, Dr. Martin said his views appeared not to be those of the majority of physicians who have dealt with DDT poisoning in humans. He said he conferred recently in Washington with Dr. Weyland J. Hayes, chief toxicologist of the U.S. Public Health Service, and Dr. Bernard Davidow of the U.S. Food and Drug Administration.

"The three of them agreed, he said, on these points: Insecticide chemicals such as chlorinated hydrocarbons and organic phosphorus are poisonous; food sprayed with them have a residue of 'varying amounts'; these poisonous residues are absorbed into the human body with the food.

" But Dr. Hayes was of the opinion that there is little proof of toxic effects in the human and therefore the danger of chronic toxicity is negligible', Dr. Martin said, ' my opinion is in direct opposition to Dr. Hayes.'

In another United Press dispatch entitled "SAYS POISONS SPRAYED ON FOODS PILE UP INSIDE EATERS", Delos Smith cites Dr. Martin again as saying:

" One-tenth part per million of DDT in the diet of rats leads to storage of about 10 to 15 parts per million of DDT in the fatty tissue of the test animal. A minimum of five parts per million of DDT produces definite pathological (disease-causing) changes in the liver of test animals.'

"'Rats fed DDT in small amounts from four to six months stored DDT in their bodies 'at a level which is 6 to 28 times the dietary intake.' These rats 'showed liver cell damage.'

"'Seven, or 28 per cent, of the positive samples (of the 25 humans tested by Dr. Martin) had five parts per million or more', he said. ' The average for all the samples was 3.5 parts per million. Age and sex seemed to have little influence on the amount of DDT accumulated in the tissue.

"More Insecticides Each Year

"In the face of all these devastating facts, DDT and other newer and more toxic insecticides are being used each year in greater and greater quantities on our food. If each year the liver damage is increased and its efficiency decreased, what will happen to the entire population in 10 to 15 years from now?

"Will a large percentage have liver dysfunction with its multiple sequellae (results), such as hyperchloesterolemia, arteriosclerosis, coronary thrombosis, cerebral hemorrhage, diabetes and all the known degenerative diseases? Will these degenerative changes start earlier in life in the next generation that begins the ingestion of these toxic chemicals at birth from mother's milk?

"These questions cannot be answered today with finality, but it is a sad commentary on our way of life, that we must spray poisonous chemicals on our food and destroy our bodies. If we hope to preserve the health of the present generation there must be some method developed to eliminate these toxic chemicals from our food that are known to produce liver damage."

In opposition to the view of government inspectors who permit the marketing of sprayed foods which contain less than the maximum amount of poison which they are permitted to contain by law, and the authorities who permit the spraying of food crops with these poisons, which are absorbed and taken up to some extent by the soil, by plants and by humans feeding on sprayed foods, Dr. Martin insists that _all_ spray poisons that come into contact with plants and trees, and which are consequently present in the vegetables and fruits they produce, are dangerous to death, and that when they do not kill us outright, they do so in a gradual manner through their cumulative effect, leading to serious chronic degenerative diseases, such as cancer, paralysis, various neurological and psychiatric disorders, etc., effects which may not manifest until ten to twenty years after initial exposure. On this point, Dr. Martin writes:

"My opinion is that even a little poison on our food is too much, especially when the poison is accumulative - when the body retains and stores it. If I came into your home at mealtime with a shaker in hand and said, 'May I sprinkle just a little poison our your food?', you'd say no - quickly and emphatically. There is no change in its toxic effect because it's put on the food before it's served. The toxic level of food should be absolutely zero. The human should have no poison in his body.

"Food free of these chemicals can be grown and is available, but not in sufficient quantity for all. Why not? "

We quote from a circular issued by the Health Guild of New York, sent with an announcement of a mass meeting devoted to the subject of "How To Eat Safely In A Poisoned World", announcing lectures by several speakers on the subjects of the chemical poisoning of food, water and cosmetics. The circular bore the title, "An Announcement of Extraordinary Significance and Vital Importance to All Health-Minded Individuals Who Wish to Protect Themselves From the Toxic Dangers of our Everyday Foods and Build a Definite Immunity and Resistance to the Health Hazards Present in their Diet.":

"A little over a year ago a Congressional Committee was convened to investigate the use of chemicals in food products. The testimony of several experts indicated that the excessive use of DDT and derivative chemicals as insecticides in the cultivation of vegetables and fruits was having a definite effect in poisoning the nation and in creating, in a cumulative manner, the toxic conditions which ultimately lay the basis for chronic diseases...diseases which now hold over 30,000,000 Americans in their agonizing grip.

"In the hearings, it was shown that over 700 different chemicals are employed in the growing, processing and preserving of foodstuffs which make up the diet of the average family, and many of these are of a nature which creates toxic effects over a period of time, if absorbed daily.

"In a recent interview released by the United Press Science Editor throughout the nation, Dr. William Coda Martin, a medical practitioner of New York, who made an intensive study of these food-poisoning chemicals, and who is an ardent advocate of organically grown vegetables, fruits, cereals, etc., made the following revealing statement. (Extracts from the United Press article above quoted are here given.) "

Dr. Biskind's Findings on Danger of Poisoning by Residues of DDT, Chlordane and Other Chlorinated Hydrocarbons in Sprayed Foods

"Substantiating Dr. Martin's views and reinforcing them by virtue of his established and recognized status as a chemical analyst, Dr. Morton Biskind of Connecticut in a press interview also issues a warning which should command the careful consideration of every health-minded person:

"'It is not generally realized how vast are the quantities of the new poisons spread over the countryside in agriculture, used as sprays and aerosol fogs in mosquito control operations and in food processing plants and retail establishments. Unfortunately, today contamination of food is virtually universal. DDT chemical poisons came into use in 1945. There has since been a number of curious changes in the incidence of certain ailments and the development of symptoms which spell out disease. A most significant feature of this situation is that both man and all his domestic animals have simultaneously been affected. These ailments are: inflammation of the liver, polio, disorders of the heart and arteries and of the gastro-intestinal tract, cancer, unusual forms of pneumonia excessive fatiguability, muscular weakness and neuropsychiatric symptoms.'

"Dr. Biskind then goes on to list a number of diseases peculiar in this period to beasts and he indicates the startling fact that none of these diseases of animals were mentioned in the Department of Agriculture's handbook on livestock issued in 1942, that is to say, before the advent of DDT and its family of chemical poisons now used in such excessive amounts in the cultivation of crops. Dr. Biskind goes on further to make this impressive revelation:

"'When DDT was released for general use, a tremendous background of toxicologic investigations had already shown beyond doubt that this chemical compound was dangerous for all animal life from insects to mammals. But it was released just the same, against the advice of these unbiased investigators. With this foreknowledge, the series of catastrophic events that followed the most intensive campaign of mass poisoning in known human history should not have surprised the experts!' "

"Louis Bromfield, the noted author and farmer, whose celebrated Malabar Farm in Ohio is in the forefront of progressive organic agriculture, stated in testimony given before the Congressional Committee of Food Intestigation, that in his opinion, when present-day medical researchers have finally admitted their failure to track down the cause of cancer, IT WOULD BE FOUND THAT THE EXCESSIVE USE OF THESE INSECTICIDES WOULD BE DEFINITELY INDICATED AS A SOURCE OF THIS DEVASTATING DISEASE WHICH NOW CLAIMS THE LIVES OF 250,000 AMERICANS EVERY YEAR!

"It is also completely convincing to note that the Hunza tribes of India who subsist entirely on products of the soil grown without chemical fertilizers (or sprays) have never had a cancer case among its people.

"Foods grown in this way are not only free from chemical poisons but also have positive values of possessing such higher mineral and vitamin content which are of primary importance for the health of the human system, besides being more flavorsome. It is common knowledge among agronomists that the excessive use of chemical fertilizers depletes the soil of health-giving minerals and vitamins, and that produce grown on soil thus contaminated and enfeebled lacks the nutritive value of organically grown crops. "

In an article, "Public Health Aspects of the New Insecticides", in the November 1953 issue of <u>The American Journal of Digestive Diseases</u>, Morton S. Biskind, M.D. presents a convincing indictment of DDT and the more highly toxic insecticides that have recently been developed. <u>Natural Living</u>, organ of Natural Food Associates, in its February 1954 issue, commenting on Dr. Biskind's article, says that it is "so impressive in volume that the reader is left with a sense of horror that science, with its immense potentialities for making man's lot safer and pleasanter, should have been so misused that, instead, his health, his mental well-being and even his life are imperiled." We now quote from an abstract of Dr. Biskind's article which appeared in this latter publication:

"Since the last war, there has been a marked increase in the incidence of certain ailments; disturbances in health, with symptoms grouped in a manner never before observed, have become common. 'A most significant feature of this situation is that both men and all his domestic animals have simultaneously been affected.' In man polio has risen sharply and there has been a striking increase in heart disease, in cancer and in pneumonia - especially in infants and children. Other conditions frequently observed are those involving excessive fatiguability and muscular weakness, diseases of the liver and obscure intestinal and nervous disorders often attributed to a new virus commonly known as virus "X".

"In 1945, DDT was released in the U.S.A. and other countries for general use. This was against the advice of investigators who found it dangerous for all forms of life. Soon after its introduction as an insecticide, it was found that insects were producing strains completely resistant to it. This led to a frantic search for ever more potent insecticides and there soon appeared chlordane, toxaphene, benzene hexachloride (BHC), lindane, heptachlor and the incredibly deadly aldrin and dieldrin. In addition, organic phosphorus compounds (closely related to the 'nerve gases' of chemical warfare) appeared on the market under the names of parathion, TEPP, HETP and others. All these compounds are lethal to man in minute doses."

In 1950, more than 200 million pounds of insecticides were used in agriculture and in the same year the Federal Food and Drug Administration announced:

"'The finding of hepatic cell alteration at dietary levels as low as 6 p.m.m. of DDT and the considerable storage of the chemical at levels that might never occur in some human diets, makes it extremely likely that the potential hazard of DDT has been under estimated.

"DDT is a delayed action poison. Due to the fact that it accumulates in the body tissues, especially in females, the repeated inhalation or ingestion of DDT constitutes a distinct health hazard. The deleterious effects are manifested principally in the liver, spleen, kidneys and spinal cord. DDT is excreted in the milk of cows and of nursing mothers after exposure to DDT sprays and after consuming food contaminated with this poison. Children and infants especially are much more susceptible to poisoning than adults. "

There is considerable evidence that new diseases among plants and animals have been directly produced by chemical fertilizers and sprays. In the case of chemical fertilizers, Keens, an English soil chemist, has shown by statistics, that the incidence of cancerous diseases among plants, animals and human beings has run parallel to the increased use of chemical fertilizers during the past century, his explanation being that these diseases resulted from aluminum poisoning, due to the action of such fertilizers in making otherwise insoluble aluminum compounds in the soil abnormally soluble, so that plants take up an excessive amount of aluminum, which they otherwise would not. This aluminum acts as a foreign poison, disturbing their metabolism ; and, in Keens' opinion, leads to the development of cancer not only in plants, but in animals and humans that feed on such aluminized vegetation.

In a similar manner, the introduction of the newly developed highly toxic sprays have led to the sudden appearance of new diseases among animals and humans. One of these is the disastrous virus "X" disease which attacks the human nervous system, as pointed out by Dr. Biskind. From the same cause, among animals there has been an increase of hoof and mouth disease, skin diseases of hogs, "blue tongue", "scrapie" and "overeating" diseases among sheep, Newcastle disease among chickens and unfamiliar liver disorders among dogs. Since none of these diseases, except hoof and mouth disease, were known prior to the introduction of these new insecticides (since they were not mentioned in the Department of Agriculture handbook on animal husbandry, "Keeping Livestock Healthy", issued in 1942), the conclusion is unavoidable that poisoning of the soil and its products on which animals feed must play an important part in the causation of these new diseases.

It is well known that , in 1945, when DDT was first introduced into agriculture, experiments conducted on animals, including rats, mice, rabbits, guinea-pigs, cats, dogs, chicks, goats, sheep, cattle, horses and monkeys, have shown that this poison produced degenerative changes in the skin, liver, gall bladder, lungs, kidneys, spleen, thyroid, adrenals, ovaries, testes, heart muscle, blood vessels, voluntary muscles, brain, spinal cord, gastro-intestinal tract and blood. Commenting on these experiments, which definitely proved that DDT was extremely harmful to mammalian life, yet which did not prevent its ever more widespread application as an insecticide in the growing of foods for human consumption, Dr. Biskind says:

"Yet, far from admitting a causal relationship so obvious that in any other field of biology it would be instantly accepted, virtually the entire apparatus of communication, lay and scientific alike, has been devoted to denying, concealing, suppressing, distorting and attempting to convert into its opposite the overwhelming evidence. Libel, slander and economic boycott have not been overlooked in this campaign. And a new principle of toxicology has, it seems, been firmly entrenched in the literature: no matter how lethal a poison may be for all other forms of animal life, if it doesn't kill human beings _instantly_ it is safe.

"In 1952, 252 million pounds of these new poisons were used in agriculture in the United States - more than 1½ lbs. for every man, woman and child in the country. This cost for all purposes amounted to 400 million dollars. In 1949, the writer has shown that exposure to DDT led to a group of symptoms which, in their entirety, had never before been known to occur. By then, however, it was occurring in hundreds of instances studied by the author, each time following a known exposure to DDT. Other investigators confirmed the author's findings and in many cases additional proof was provided by the discovery of DDT in the body fat of the patient."

Ignorant of the true cause of this new strange disease, medical science ascribed it to a new virus and called it virus "X" disease. Dr. F.L. Mickle, writing in the Connecticut Health Bulletin for January 1952, says:

"Virus diseases, which appear to be increasing, are coming to the foreground. They are of much greater importance in the State than formerly. For instance, almost every person you meet on the street or in the homes of your friends speaks at one time of having had the 'virus that's going around.'

Dr. Biskind points out that in addition to these new so-called "virus" diseases, the incidence of polio has more than doubled since 1946. Since then, rather than occurring spasmodically, as it did in the past, polio has remained epidemic year after year. And while the disease was formerly confined largely to children, now more and more adults are acquiring it. Why this change?

It is Dr. Biskind's view that just as DDT poisoning is the cause of the mysterious virus "X" disease, so it is also largely responsible for the modern increase of polio, another nerve disease.

The fact that polio epidemics are more common during the summer months would indicate that, since at this time of the year more vegetables and fruits are consumed, there is greater intake of poisonous insecticide residues than at other seasons, these poisons affecting the spinal cord and causing the symptoms of polio. In evidence of such a possibility, Dr. Biskind points out that American troops in the Phillipines and elsewhere in the Far East, who used vast quantities of DDT as an insecticide, had a high incidence of polio, whereas it was extremely low in the surrounding native population. In Israel, before DDT was widely used, only one or two cases of polio occurred monthly in the entire nation, whereas in 1950, after it had been introduced and widely used, 1600 cases were listed - more than one case per thousand.

In addition to polio, another disease which has increased alarmingly in recent years, and which Dr. Biskind believes is to some extent caused or aggravated by DDT poisoning, is heart disease. The Federal Food and Drug Administration has reported that DDT produces "an excessive excitability of the cardiac muscle", causing irregular beating of the muscle fibers of the heart ventricles - a serious and often fatal condition.

Recently we have heard much about a possible connection between cancer of the lungs and the use of tobacco. Yet, about twenty years ago, cancer of the lungs was a comparatively rare disease, even among long-term intemperate smokers. Why the sudden appearance of this disease? Dr. Biskind traces this to the fact that in growing tobacco, the crop is sprayed with several of the DDT series of compounds, as well as with organic phosphorus compounds; and among the insecticides used are chlordane, toxaphene and lindane, all highly dangerous. The residues of these poisons vaporize in the smoke. They were not present in tobacco smoke twenty years ago. In Dr. Biskind's opinion, the intake of these poisons is a probable cause of the present increasing prevalence of lung cancer among smokers.

Another disease that has increased tremendously in recent times is inflammation of the liver, whose rise in frequency in the general population since 1945 is without parallel and involves all age groups, including infants. Dr. Biskind points out the interesting fact that this disease, within recent years, has become increasingly common among animals, such as cattle, dogs and other farm animals, spreading among them coincidently with its increase among humans. Here, again, we have reason to suspect the newly developed highly toxic insecticides as being responsible. On this point, Dr. Biskind says:

"It would be a most remarkable coincidence if several entirely different hepatic infective agents, each specific to a different animal species, arose simultaneously. Human inectious hepatitis is not transmissable to dogs or cattle...without exception, however, every one of the chlorinated hydrocarbon insecticides is a liver poison."

From the facts presented in this chapter one must conclude that the entire American public is now being subjected to a constant barrage of newly invented super-poisons which, while ostensibly designed to destroy insects that attack food crops, are at the same time ruining the vital organs and bringing on serious chronic degenerative diseases that shorten the life-span of humans. The most dangerous thing about these poisonous sprays is that they tend to accumulate in the soil; and some of them are very difficult to get rid of, resisting even the eroding influence of rainfall. Tests have shown that some of them were present in soils at near their original concentration even years after they were sprayed on growing crops. This would mean that even if plants are not sprayed, they may take up insecticide residues from contaminated soil, resulting from the spraying of previous crops, and communicate these poisons to the INTERIOR of vegetables. Spray poisons may also find their way into the sap of plants and trees and thus be communicated to the INTERIOR of vegetables and fruits by direct leaf absorption of sprays applied to their surface. That this may occur is indicated by the practice of direct plant feeding by spraying nutrients on their leaves. That the entire American population, in this way, is subjected to mass poisoning, which cannot be avoided by washing or peeling vegetables and fruits, which fail to remove the toxic spray residues they contain within them, is indicated by Dr. Biskind as follows:

"Exposure to this whole group of compounds is now universal in the United States and it appears that few persons escape storage of these toxic agents in the body fat. DDT has been found to occur in human fact in all but a few of the cases examined. It has been found in mother's milk. As little as 3 parts per million has been found to be detrimental, but in the fat of DDT handlers as much as 291 p.p.m. has been found. In a group of volunteers from widely scattered sections of the United States, the average concentration was 6.41 p.p.m., with the highest 68 p.p.m."

Investigators for the U.S. Public Health Service reported in September 1952: "Presumably the DDT occurring in the fat of individuals of the general population arises mainly through the contamination of a number of common foodstuffs". As we have already pointed out, the most tragoc and threetening aspect of the problem of the danger of some of the new highly potent chlorinated hydrocarbons is that once they are sprayed on a growing crop, the soil becomes poisoned for years, so that the poison will reappear in future crops planted on the same land; and it will be impossible to get rid of it, whether crops are sprayed or not. Such soil poisoning by insecticide residues has been noticed in apple orchards in the State of Washington, where sufficient arsenic accumulated in the soil so that grass cannot grow. Tests have shown that the new chlorinated hydrocarbons are far more tenacious either than arsenic or DDT in their capacity to remain in the soil. They are gradually poisoning American farmlands and rendering them unfit to produce safe and healthful foods. This lends an entirely different picture to the seriousness of the spraying menace. Formerly it was a question whether to spray or not to spray, in the former case, foods being considered contaminated by spray residues, while in the latter case they were unsprayed and therefore safe to eat. But with the soil being contaminated with insecticide poisons, they will be present in the interior of vegetables and fruits, whether they are sprayed or not. The only way to obtain safe, unpoisoned foods under such conditions will be to not grow them on lands on which previous sprayed crops were raised, but only on new virgin land.

Not only do these new powerful insecticides poison the soil of our farms, but also the air which city dwellers breathe, since they are constantly exposed to them. These terribly potent poisons attack us on all sides in modern civilized life. They are vaporized by heating devices in homes, restaurants and food stores, as well as in public buildings, to destroy flies, mosquitoes and other insects. They are incorporated into paints and wall paper, as well as floor wax. They are used to mothproof almost every variety of textile. They are sprayed and painted on every conceivable surface in homes and public institutions. According to Dr. Biskind, dangerous residues may persist on treated surfaces for very long periods, slowly poisoning those exposed to them. While, years ago, cases of lead and arsenic poisoning have been not uncommon, as a result of exposure to newly painted walls and wallpaper colored by arsenic compounds, today the danger is graver, since these new poisons are more likely to contaminate the air and to be inhaled.

But the chief source of insecticide poisoning is in the form of sprayed foods. On this subject, Dr. Biskind writes: " Today, contamination of food is virtually universal. Even if the farmer does not use the new insecticides, it is rare for a food to escape contact with insecticides in storage, shipment, processing plants, wharehouses and stores. In Texas, in the year 1950, every sample of meat and milk purchases by investigators in the open market was found to contain DDT, rising to the appalling figure of 68.5 p.p.m. in a sample of fat meat.

"It is claimed that without the use of these new insecticides there would not be enough food to go around. But it has been shown by a number of agricultural workers that these virulent poisons, in the long run, are actually determiental to both crop production and the prevention of disease carried by insects...Everywhere that DDT has been used for any length of time, strains of insects, both those that attack crops as well as flies, mosquitoes and lice, have become resistant, not only to DDT but to related compounds as well."

In confirmation of the view expressed above by Dr. Biskind, Pickett and De Bach have both reported that DDT and related poisons, used for spraying orchards, actually increase the menace of insect pests by building up insecticide resistance in them, while at the same time killing natural predators of harmful insects. On this point Dr. Biskind writes: "The futility of the chemical approach ...is perhaps no better illustrated than by the fact that after seven or eight years of the most intensive imaginable poison campaign, virtually the entire 'bread basket' area of the United States was blanketed in 1953 with army worms that destroyed vast areas of food crops...It was admitted by the U.S.D.A. that further chemical attack was fruitless, although the same department then released the extremely toxic dieldrin for use against them!"

Chlordane, the New Super Killer

As dangerous as DDT is, chlordane is far worse. In a report published by the U.S. Printing Office in 1951, A.J. Lehman of the Federal Food and Drug Administration said:

"In my opinion, chlordane is one of the most toxic insecticides we have to deal with...It penetrates the skin very readily. Therefore, anyone handling it could be poisoned...It is very toxic to the liver and kidneys...I would put chlordane four to five times more poisonous than DDT...I would hesitate to eat food that had any chlordane on it whatsoever...It is our opinion that chlordane has no place in the food industry where even the remotest opportunity for contamination exists. We have not been able to maintain pigeons in a small room that was treated with chlordane even after a thorough scrubbing with strong alkali and subsequent airing for several weeks."

Yet in spite of this official opinion on the extreme toxicity of chlordane, in the *Proceedings of the American Chemical Society*, 1949, p.18, Holmes and Salathe say: "Experience has shown, within the baking industry, that DDT and chlordane can be applied safely, in 5 to 2 per cent solutions respectively...The application must be so general that there are few, if any, areas that insects might travel over which have not been treated."

In 1952, a popular publication of immense circulation advised its readers to apply chlordane to floors, base boards, sinks, under refrigerators, to mattresses, wallpapers, rugs, clothes-closets and clothing. The following statement by Dr. Biskind indicates how misleading this advice is. In a hospital in which chlordane is applied routinely in the kitchen and food storeroom for roach control, an epidemic of hepatitis has persisted among the resident nursing staff for three years. This disorder has been considered "infectious", yet despite adequate epidemiologic precautions the cases continued to appear. Chlordane was still in use.

Formerly it was arsenic and lead poisoning; yesterday it was DDT poisoning; and today it is chlordane poisoning. An interesting case of chlordane poisoning is recorded in the February 1954 issue of Natural Living. It is the case of Harry Pagoda, a New Yorker who got chlordane poisoning while in the exterminator business. Through an organic diet, composed of unsprayed, organically grown foods, on which he lived for three years, he recovered; and today says that he never felt better in his life. He tells his own story:

"I have been on an organic diet about three years. I was made sick by chlordane in exterminating work. It is ten times more toxic than DDT according to my doctor.

"I had paralysis of the face, tremors in the ankles, knees, legs and internal tremors; violent, continuous pains in the head. Pains in my spine and shoulders, bounding pains in various parts of the body, and intermittent pains.

"Both arms would be numb and both legs, simultaneously. My hands would be paralyzed intermittently for an hour and then they would open up after being closed. At the beginning I had a violent pain in my throat that would last a couple of hours and then it would vanish.

"My present doctor diagnosed my trouble as chlordane poisoning in September 1949. In the beginning he said to peel all vegetables and to eat none that could not be peeled, but later he said that it would not be sufficient; that vegetables grown and sprayed with DDT or chlordane or any of these chlorinated hydrocarbon insecticides would contain much insecticide in the crop, whatever it was, even in tobacco. I was a cigar smoker and he told me to stop smoking. He put me on an organic diet about 3 years ago.

"My doctor told me to stay away from any place that had been sprayed with such chlorinated hydrocarbon insecticides, any place, building or store, because dust in the air picks up the residues, even a year or so later, unless the place has been painted.

"I saw a sharp improvement in my health after being on an organic diet about a year and have improved gradually but steadily since. ...Today I have a terrific amount of vitality."

704 Different Chemicals in Our Foods

Investigations by the Federal Food and Drug Administration showed that 704 different chemicals are used regularly in the nation's food processing, and that of these, only 426 are known to be "safe". (We may ask how any chemical added to foods can be truly "safe". Though it may not produce any immediate harmful effects that are apparent, what about its gradual cumulative effects that may not manifest until years later. Chemical fertilizer residues in foods are of this type.)

Among 278 chemicals added to foods that are known to be definitely poisonous is the group of toxic insecticide chemicals found in practically all vegetables and fruits sold in American public markets. The others are also harmful, since the human body can assimilate and utilize only organically combined minerals, but cannot metabolize in-organic minerals in the form of chemicals, which, when they do not poison or kill one outright, produce slow cumulative injury to vital organs. On this subject, Representative John L. Delaney of New York, head of a committee which has studied the question of fortifying legislation to protect the public from poisonous pesticides and chemical additives in foods and cosmetics, says:

"Our food supply is being doctored by hundreds of new chemicals whose safety has not yet been established. Many of these chemicals were developed during and after World War II. Most of them may prove harmless, but enough have been proven dangerous, and even deadly so as to make us wonder if our health is threatened...The growing number of mental diseases (may be related to) the many new chemicals used in our food...Doctors testifying before the house committee have stated there may be some connection between these new chemicals and the increase in such diseases as cancer, polio and the mysterious virus "X".

In an article, "Poison by the Plateful", in the March 1954 issue of *Organic Gardening and Farming*, M.C. Goldman writes:

"Starting with the very growing of crops, there has evolved a startling increase in chemicalization since, let us say, 1938 - the last time <u>any</u> attempt was made to moderate our Food and Drug laws. Chemical treatments are more and more being applied to seeds - and how most of these influence the resulting product is as much or more undetermined as the effects of various applications to our foods in any other stage. Another recent crop innovation is the applying of several different hormones to modify growth and ripening. Again, the results may be accepted in terms of plant control, but they are unknown in terms of long-range human effects, particularly with such hormones designed to retard or speed growth.

"Next consider the increasing mass of chemicals being applied to crops right after harvesting and during periods of storage. Economically, they aim at better keeping quality, resistance to after-harvest disease and insect infestation - but from a health and nutrition standpoint they haven't all been shown safe. On the contrary, a recent farm journal - which discusses stored grain treatment with DDT, methoxychlor and the newer chemical with the tongue-twisting name pyrethrum-peperonyl butoxide - makes a cautioning note that chlordane, a common insecticide enjoying wide usage today, is no longer considered safe for this purpose and 'should under no circumstances be used to treat granaries or grain bins'. We simply wonder just how safe many of these other treatments really are.

"Mentioning insecticides in general usually brings DDT to mind - along with its since-developed spray cousins. DDT saw wartime use as a typhus and malaria preventive, when the danger of injury to troops was considered less than the danger from these diseases. However, the evidence has since been clear that cows sprayed with DDT or fed silage treated with it can secrete it in the butterfat of their milk in dangerous amounts. The American Medical Association's committee on pesticides has reported that chronic poisoning may result from the ingestion of small amounts of DDT over a period of time, and the safe tolerance level is unknown."

Dr. Mobbs' Studies on Spray Poisoning

The noted news commentator, Drew Pearson, in a recent news release, described a hearing before the House Interstate and Foreign Commerce Committee, at which Dr. Mobbs, a prominent North Carolina physician, after five years of study of the problem, boldly stated that the American people are now being poisoned on a mass scale by some of the more newly developed highly toxic insecticides, in comparison with which the old-fashioned sprays are relatively mild and inocuous. One of these is benzene hexachloride, which was found in tests to produce abnormal, cancer-like cell growth.

Dr. Mobbs' investigations commenced as a result of observing the death of a child living in a home adjacent to an insecticide mixing plant, who suddenly died in convulsions. As a result of experiments with animals which also died in convulsions, Dr. Mobbs concluded that the cause of death was ingestion of insecticide dust present in the air. To the same cause he attributed a strange virus-like disease that was rampant in the town.

Dr. Mobbs therefore appealed to congressmen to pass laws establishing stricter regulation of the use of dangerous insecticides, such as benzene hexachloride, which is used not only to spray fruits and vegetables, but in vaporizing devices used in homes and restaurants.

His appeal, however, fell on deaf ears, for instead of adapting his recommendations, the committee boosted a bill endorsed by the insecticide companies that would leave it up to the manufacturers to test their own pesticides and to submit their findings to the government. The Federal Food and Drug Administration would then decide, on the basis of the manufacturer's _own_ report, how large a dose of poison could be given to the public.

Due to the widespread use of insecticides in North Carolina, one of the largest packers of baby foods stopped buying foods in this state, since tests of North Carolina vegetables showed a heavy residue of DDT and other insecticides. Looking elsewhere for safe sources of vegetables and other foods he required for the manufacture of baby foods, this manufacturer was forced to abandon the search - for he found that all vegetables grown and sold in this country, in sufficient quantities for his needs, contained smaller or larger amounts of insecticide residues, in many cases, enough to produce toxic effects. Finally he was forced to use such poisoned vegetables, even though he knew that they were harmful to babies. Safe, unsprayed, unpoisoned foods, he found, were unavailable in this most advanced and most "civilized" of all nations on earth. This clearly indicates the crying need for organically grown foods free from poisons, not only for babies, but for everyone.

In an article, "Insecticides in North Carolina", in the July 1953 issue of _Prevention_, we read: "In almost every county of the state's big fertilizer belt in the East and Piedmont, there are instances of farmers and animals dying from insect spraying - often in convulsions. State College researchers, just beginning to check on the possible deadly effects of these poisons on human beings, have found that two of the three people tested in postmortems showed DDT in their tissue. (On a national basis, the Food and Drug Administration, testing 75 samples of human tissue, found DDT in 62 cases.) A scientist in Dallas, suspecting its presence in most foods on the market today, bought meat and milk at random in Texas markets, and discovered DDT in all these commodities he bought."

Benzine hexachloride was developed by the Germans as a wartime poison gas. It is considered to be very deadly. Besides being used as an insecticide for the spraying of vegetables and fruits, it is now used in every progressive restaurant, where it is vaporized, to kill insects that may come in. It is called lindane. Since it has never been thoroughly tested, there are no government regulations concerning its use. Nevertheless it is a powerful killer, as shown by the observations of Dr. Mobbs:

Another newly developed insecticide which is highly poisonous is parathion. This insecticide is used everywhere today. Last spring parathion killed two men almost at the same time, as they worked their tobacco fields at Latta, S.C. and Tabor City, S.C. This insecticide was also developed in Germany. Dr. Mobbs has gathered records of one hundred deaths in this country due to parathion and benzine hexachloride. No one knows, however, how many other persons have become sick or been afflicted with some chronic ailment, dying prematurely at a later date, from exposure to this toxic substance. On this subject, Dr. Mobbs writes: "One of the great dangers is the residual effect from eating foods contaminated with DDT and other poisons. They seem to build up in the fatty tissues of the body. We know that much, but precious little more. "

Prevention comments as follows on Dr. Mobbs' observations: "The young doctor is not talking about isolated cases or remote dangers. The newspapers have been literally filled with recurring cases of deaths from these poisons in the past few years. Some Carolina examples: Five cows dead at Lumber Ridge; 100 chickens at Maxton, seven pigs at Clio, S.C. Dozens of persons, chiefly farm workers, have died under circumstances indicating they were poisoned by insecticides.

"Mobbs, despite congressional interest, is not optimistic. 'The chemical industry put up $120,000.00 last winter to suppress unfavorable publicity about insecticides', he says...Mobbs is outraged by some things which have happened to him - though he is not surprised by loss of some of his practice. One man from the Federal Security Agency came to see him, he says, and warned him to tone down his squawks about insecticides. He pointed out to Mobbs, the doctor said, that Deutsch, a New York writer who exposed some insecticides as deadly and beyond control, 'was taken care of'. "

What can be done to stem the insecticide menace? Will government regulations, laws and prohibitions solve the problem? The answer is that they will not. So long as crops are attacked by insects, insecticides will be resorted to - for otherwise the public will have no food to eat. The solution of the problem is to remove the basic <u>cause</u> of the insect pests, rather than to combat them directly. This cause, we are convinced, is a wrong method of chemical fertilization, which creates weakened and unhealthy plants which lack resistance to insect marauders, which seem to play the role of parasites that attack only defective plants that have been improperly nourished, so helping to get rid of them. Experiments have shown that when plants are properly fertilized, with an abundance of powdered rocks that supply all essential trace minerals, and without chemicals, they are not attacked by insects and so need no spraying. Many years ago, Dr. Julius Hensel in Germany and Sampson Morgan in England proved this fact. Through a system of natural soil regeneration and fertilization which they developed, without the use of animal or chemical fertilizers, they produced vegetables and fruits that possessed absolute immunity to insect pests as well as diseases of all kinds. This new method of agriculture will be explained in our forthcoming work. "Super

Chapter Two

ADDITIONAL EVIDENCE CONCERNING THE DAILY, EVER-PRESENT PRESENCE OF INSECTICIDE RESIDUES IN FOODS

John Dendy, head of the Analytical Chemistry Division of the Texas Research Foundation at Renner, Texas, found that all meat and milk purchased at retail stores in the neighborhood contained DDT, which was used on farms in the area. The degree of contamination ranged from 3.10 parts per million of DDT in lean meat to 68.55 parts per million in fat meat. In milk the contamination ranged from less than .5 parts of DDT per million to 13.83 parts per million.

In the case of corn and sunflowers sprayed with chlorinated hydrocarbons, these were found in the grains and seeds in unchanged form, having been absorbed from the soil by the roots of the plant. The rate of absorption was found to be cumulative, the degree of contamination increasing with each spraying. DDT, toxaphene, chlordane, BHC, methoxychlor and aldrin were the insecticides used. They were found to accumulate in the soil and to become higher and higher in concentration, both in the soil and in foods grown thereon, as time went on.

In the case of milk, it was found that DDT was present therein even months after the spraying of cows was discontinued, indicating that the insecticide was stored in the animal's body and contaminated the milk that it produced at a later date.

Prevention lists the following "horror stories" of people killed or made ill by exposure to sprays. These are sample headlines: "Girl Dies After Eating (Sprayed) Peaches" (the other four children escaped death but were violently ill), "Potato Growers Warned on Use of Insecticides", "Industrial Intoxication Due to Pentachlorophenol " (an insecticide and fungicide), "Disastrous Results in Peach Orchard Following Use of Benzene Hexachloride and DDT", "Insecticide (sodium selenate) Found to Cause Sterility and Loss of Hair", "Pheasants Poisoned by Eating Grain Treated to Prevent Smut", "Six Fatal Cases of Carbon Tetrachloride Poisoning", "Twenty-nine Are Stricken After Working in Tobacco Field". "And so on and on through a tragic story of illness and death from exposure to poison sprays either in manufacturing them, in spraying fruits and vegetables, or in eating them after they have been sprayed. "

Since insects tend to become resistant to insecticide chemicals, it is necessary to develop newer and more powerful ones; and so the death race of man against insects goes on- the insects gaining immunity to man's newly developed poisons, while he increasingly succumbs to them. On this point, *Prevention*, in its March 1952 issue, from which the above was quoted, says: "In other words, in a never-ending lethal cycle, we must produce ever more powerful poisons, to which whole species of insects will eventually become resistant, making it necessary to douse them with still more powerful stuff. A writer of horror stories might well imagine the situation a century from now, if this tendency continues unchecked. We will have a world full of insects which our own insecticides will have made resistant to the point where no poison will kill them and a race of men subject to countless new diseases because of eating, breathing, and handling these poisons. And we will have a topsoil poisoned to the point where nothing will grow on it.

According to Dr. James A. Curren, Entomologist of the American Museum of Natural History, DDT sprayed on peach trees actually increased the number of pests by killing parasites which controlled the peach moth. He also found that DDT stays in the soil for at least two years; and since it is not readily soluble in water it doesn't seem to be readily washed down into the subsoil by rainfall, but remains in the topsoil. Dr. Curran says: "That reminds us of the results we had with certain arsenicals used in the orchards out West. After many years of this there was so much in the soil, it contaminated the grass and cattle died eating it. DDT is essentially much stronger than these arsenicals...A lot more experimenting should be done before turning every man and boy loose in the open with a spray gun."

In the Northwest apple-producing belt so much lead arsenate is applied to the trees that there may be as much as 1800 pounds reaching the soil of an acre of land in a ten-year period. The soil becomes so saturated with arsenic that finally even grass will not grow. What about the arsenate that the roots of the apple trees take up and communicate, through the sap, to the INTERIOR of the apples – this amount increasing year after year, as the soil becomes increasingly saturated with arsenate of lead? Consumers Research, in May - 1949 - issue, comments: "This is surely an interesting if somewhat alarming illustration of the dilemma which man gets into in his attempts to improve on nature and to worst the natural enemies of farm produce in the growing of crops."

In an article, "The Widespread Dangers of Insecticides", in the May 1952 issue of *Prevention*, we read: "Now that many new insecticide sprays are being used, more recently discovered and more powerful than lead, arsenic and DDT, there is cause for more alarm than ever before. Our food is continually contaminated with poisons so new that there has been little time to do any experimenting on the damage they may do to human beings, animals, insects, plants or to the soil itself.

"A warning on the dangers of Parathion is headlined 'Insecticide Poisoning Warning Given! In the article which follows, a state health commissioner warns all readers to avoid working in fields sprayed with parathion for at least five days after the spray has been applied. The warning was issued after a number of farm workers had been admitted to hospitals, seriously poisoned. An article in The American Practitioner for January 1951 discloses six deaths during the past year from parathion poisoning, along with a 'number of non-fatal accidents.'

In the New York Herald-Tribune for April 15, 1951, a warning is issued concerning the use of chlordane, BHC and parathion, as follows: "Chlordane and BHC taint the taste of fruits and vegetables. BHC, applied to the soil to control wireworms, gave off an off-flavor to the following three crops of potatoes." The article further warned that these insecticides "are extremely dangerous to humans. They are probably too dangerous to use in the garden or to have around the house." (But what about the danger of soil contamination with these poisons and their effect on future crops?)

Quoting again from the May 1952 issue of Prevention, we read: "One of the most frightening aspects of the contamination of foods and soil by insecticides is that it is going on all the time, twenty-four hours a day, without any private citizen being given an opportunity to do anything about it. He has no way of knowing whether the fruit and vegetables he buys at the corner grocery have been poisoned by sprays. If a member of his family becomes ill from eating the poison, there is nothing he can do but protest to the County Health Department which will probably refer it to the State Health Department, which will issue a warning cautioning farmers in the use of this particular poison.

"Even more frightening is the prospect of the illnesses these poisons may be storing up in our bodies which we will not know about for many years to come. Lead poisoning, for instance, sometimes does not produce any symptoms for as long as ten years. Then its effect may be to lower the body's resistance to some disease or other, whose sudden onslaught in a supposedly healthy person will be mysterious and hard to trace back to the lead poison.

"In the case of the newer insecticides, even the scientists who made them do not know what potentialities these poisons may have for lowering our resistance to all kinds of diseases. Yet we go on using them, casually and carelessly. Why should it be that in America, with our high standard of living, our many health and research foundations, our careful pure food and drug regulations, we should be plagued with diseases unknown in Europe and Asia? Might it not be explained by the simple fact that in those countries poisons are not distributed on a national scale, for any and every farmer to use, with or without reading the label?"

In an article in the Cleveland Plain Dealer of September 9, 1951, Louis Bromfield writes about the work of the Congressional committee under the direction of Representative Delaney, for the purpose of securing information concerning the whole matter of the poisons contaminating our foods, and, if possible, to recommend legislation to protect us "from a menace suffered by no other people in the world." Mr. Bromfield's words are eloquent:

"The committee investigations have given rise to one of the most extraordinary smear campaigns in our history. Mr. Delaney has been blackguarded and those who testified that we know nothing of the effects of the strange new poisons have been called liars, fools and virtually threatened with blackmail. The campaign is traceable to exactly one source - the giant chemical manufacturers who make millions each year out of the tons of poisons ued in the growing and processing of American food. Whether the responsible executives of these companies are aware of the facts or not I do not know, but I suggest that they inform themselves."

Chapter Three
POISON ON TAP : THE CHEMICAL AND METALLIC CONTAMINATION
OF DRINKING WATER

In the last chapter we spoke of the poisoning of our food supply by highly toxic chemicals in the form of insecticides. In this chapter we shall discuss the poisoning of our water supply by chlorine, aluminum, fluorine and dissolved pipe metals. It is clear that if we use safe, organically grown foods, but use ordinary chemicalized water, the latter will undo the beneficial effects of the former. Chemical-free water is as important for health as chemical-free food. In the October 1953 issue of Prevention, its editor, J.I.Rodale, writes as follows on this subject:

"Drinking water has come in for a large share of attention on Prevention pages, since the campaign for fluoridating water has gone into full swing. But there are other angles to good water aside from water fluoridation. For instance, did you ever write to your water company and ask them what chemicals go into the stuff that comes out of your water faucets? It might amaze you to find out just how many are put in. Most cities and towns use chlorine and we have shown in past issues of Prevention that no one has ever done a complete survey of all the bad effects on health that might result from drinking chlorinated water over a period of years. We have also reported on a number of cases of allergies, hives, asthma and so forth that we have shown were caused by chlorinated water.

"And speaking of drinking water, if you have a water softener, we don't advise drinking or cooking with water that has been through a softener. Chemicals in the softener remove some minerals from the water and put others in their place. The calcium is removed, for instance, for calcium is what makes water 'hard'. In its place you are likely to get sodium, which is especially undesirable if you are trying to stay on a low-sodium diet. If you're planning to have a softener put in, arrange to have it on the hot water line only, so that the cold water you use for drinking and cooking will be uncontaminated with the dubious chemicals introduced by the water softener."

In the March 1954 issue of Organic Gardening and Farming, Rodale again writes: "Our drinking water has chlorine in it and in a recent issue of the Journal of the American Medical Association, it was admitted that no tests had ever been made to test the effect of chlorine on either man or animal. And in this connection, an organic gardener should never use chlorinated water to sprinkle on his soil. In many municipal systems alum and sulphur dioxide are used along with the chlorine - with what effect no one can tell. "

The Menace of Chlorination

Chlorine is the poison gas used in World War I, which proved so deadly that its use was prohibited in World War II. Instead of being let loose on the enemy, this poison gas was, however, administered to the civilian population by adding it to their water supply, so that it was received through the mouth rather than through the nose, and in sufficiently dilute proportion to disguise its poisonous nature and hide its harmful effects, which, being cumulative, are unnoticed.

When the practice of chlorinating city water supplies was first introduced, there was considerable objection to it by the medical profession, which traced various pathological conditions to this cause - just as today there is a similar opposition to the practice of fluoridation. But as time passed, the opposition died down; and chlorination became a universal practice in every city and town in the country. It is now being considered as a perfectly harmless practice. But is this really so? Could a chemical which has proven so poisonous when inhaled in gaseous form be entirely harmless when taken in liquid form, by adding it to our drinking water? And is a substance which is known to be a deadly poison in high concentration entirely harmless when taken in low concentration?

A number of cases have been reported where heavily chlorinated swimming pools proved injurious to swimmers and to fish and other living organisms emersed in such water. New England newspapers recently reported a case where a score or so of children were violently ill from chlorine poisoning by bathing in a swimming pool whose water had been heavily chlorinated. While the gasping, choking children were given artificial respiration in a hospital, authorities investigated the cause of the accident. They found that a filter had backfired, so that an extra amount of chlorine had been released into the water of the pool. It was surmised that the children had either swallowed some of the heavily chlorinated water or were simply overcome by the fumes. They turned blue and dizzy and nearly choked. An overdose of chlorine was considered to be the cause of the poisoning.

Commenting on this case, *Prevention* says: "But how much is an overdose for each individual cell of our bodies when you and I drink chlorinated water daily, year after year? We suspect that practically all *Prevention* readers who live in cities or towns are drinking chlorinated water. As an experiment it might be worth while to buy enough bottled spring water to last the family a week or two. Use this water exclusively for drinking and cooking and see whether there is an improvement in any complaints members of the family may have - such as hives, asthma or some other allergic disturbance."

There is considerable medical evidence that chlorinated water has a disease-producing effect on the consumer. Dr. Clarke of London made a special study of the question, and found that chlorine added to drinking water produced definite pathological conditions. These usually pass unnoticed when insufficient chlorine is taken, but are marked when the concentration of chlorine in drinking water increases, especially in allergic individuals. The following symptoms were traced by Dr. Clarke to chlorine poisoning: colds, catarrhs, acute rheumatism, inflamed and ulcerated mouth, malignant pustules, dry yellow and shriviled skin, etc.

The January 1953 issue of *Prevention* published an article, "Chlorine the Villain", which referred to the studies on chlorine poisoning from drinking water conducted by M.J. Gutmann, M.D. in the *Journal of Allergy* in the November 1944 issue. A case was reported of giant hives in an English officer stationed in Jerusalem. Tests showed that over forty different foods tried failed to produce symptoms of allergy, nor was it of bacterial origin. The disease disappeared only when the officer was transferred from Jerusalem to other stations where he drank mineral water, rather than the chlorinated city water of Jerusalem. As soon as he returned to Jerusalem and drank the chlorinated water, the hives promptly reappeared.

Dr. Gutmann refers to another case where chlorinated water was the cause of asthma and functional colitis. When the patient was put on distilled water exclusively for three days, both disorders disappeared. But when just one drop of a chlorine compound was added to the drinking water, the asthma and colitis promptly returned. Dr. Gutmann reports that he has had other patients who contracted hives from addition of even the smallest amount of chlorine to their drinking water. One case was that of a woman of 28 who had hives all her life, and who tried all kinds of diets without avail. Finally someone thought of changing her drinking water. As soon as the chlorinated drinking water was discontinued, the hives disappeared within a few days. But when she returned to the use of chlorinated water, the eruptions appeared within a short time.

Addition of chlorine to city water supplies leads to the formation of a certain quantity of hydrochloric acid in the water, which makes it a better solvent of pipe metals. For this reason chlorinated water tends to take up larger amounts of metal from the pipes through which it passes than non-chlorinated water. It is a fact that hydrochloric acid combines with zinc, a constituent of galvanized pipes, forming zinc chloride, a poisonous substance. Galvanized pipes are the kind most commonly used today. Iron, another constituent of such pipes, is also acted on by hydrochloric acid, forming iron chloride. Iron rust is another source of metallic contamination of piped water. Use of such metal-containing water, day after day, year after year, should lead to harmful cumulative effects, even though the small amount of metal ingested daily may not produce any immediate symptoms. However, this is not true in the case of lead pipes, which are known to have produced many cases of lead poisoning, affecting the spinal cord and leading to paralysis and other symptoms, the frequency of which in former years led to the replacement of lead pipes by the galvanized ones now in common use. (However, lead is still used by plumbers in pipe joints and fittings; and a certain amount of lead might in this way enter into the water.)

Metallic Poisoning From Water Pipes

That metallic poisoning by use of water flowing through metal pipes is a real health hazard, though generally ignored today, was widely recognized by the medical profession some decades ago, when lead pipes were in common use. At that time, cases of lead poisoning from drinking water flowing through lead pipes were frequently cited in medical literature. In fact such cases were so frequently mentioned that public conscience was awakened concerning the menace of lead pipes, with the result that their use was discontinued; and galvanized pipes were used instead. But are galvanized pipes perfectly safe?

Clear evidence that they are not are the many cases where people replaced galvanized pipes by copper pipes, often at considerable expense. If galvanized pipes were perfectly satisfactory, and were 100% insoluble, there would be no need for such replacement. The fact that they were replaced would indicate that they did contaminate the water flowing through them.

When lead pipes were in common use, while cases of acute lead poisoning, leading to such symptoms as paralysis occurred only in isolated instances, more serious is the widespread subacute chronic lead poisoning that affected entire populations. Evidence that this was so is the phrase "normal lead" that appeared in medical literature of the time, referring to the lead deposits found in the bones, spinal cord and other parts of the bodies of practically all postmortems examined, this lead, it was admitted, since it was not a normal physiological mineral, being a foreign impurity, whose origin was traced to the use of drinking water flowing through lead pipes, foods cooked in lead-containing white enamelware, exposure to the fumes of white lead paint, absorption of lead through the skin of the hands by contact with such paint, etc. Another source of lead poisoning in former times was the use of lead fillings in teeth. A certain amount of lead was dissolved by the saliva; and thus the lead fillings slowly poisoned the body. Recognition of this danger led to the replacement of lead fillings by amalgam (silver-mercury) fillings, as the kind most commonly put into teeth by dentists today, especially when the patient cannot afford more expensive gold fillings. But are amalgam fillings entirely safe? We shall present evidence below to prove that they are not.

The word "plumber", etymologically, means one who works with lead, since lead was the metal most commonly used for plumbing years ago. The discontinuance of the use of lead pipes, due to their known harmful effect on health has not, however, done away with sources of lead poisoning in modern life. Among these are the following: lead insecticide residues in fruits and vegetables that were sprayed with arsenate of lead, lead present in most enamelware, especially white, lead in water pipe joints and fittings, lead used to seal tin cans, lead in white rubber nipples, lead in milk that has been collected or stored in lead pails and milk cans, etc.

If lead, dissolved by water flowing through lead pipes and contaminating such water is recognized to be a health hazard, what about zinc and iron dissolved from galvanized pipes? Are these metals in our drinking water entirely harmless? The fact that these metals do not produce such dramatic effects as the paralysis that results from lead poisoning does not mean that they are harmless. What about the cumulative effects of these metals when ingested each day in small quantities, year after year?

The common practice of letting the water from a kitchen faucet run for a while before drinking it (usually rinsing one's glass a few times to let some time pass by), is probably a product of an often unconscious realization that the water which first comes out - the water that has stood in water pipes the longest time and which consequently had greatest opportunity to dissolve metals from these pipes - is not as desirable as the freely flowing water which emerges after the faucet has been turned on for a while, which had less opportunity to dissolve and take up metals from pipes. This practice of letting the water run before drinking it is in itself a testimonial that drinking water does contain metals dissolved from pipes, and that such metals are harmful and should be avoided. Concerning the fact that metals dissolved from water pipes and present in drinking water may be a cause of disease, P.L. Kourenoff, in his *Oriental Folk Remedies*, says:

"In childhood days the author often listened to stories told by his family doctor, I.N. Vinogradoff, who sent hundreds of patients of all ages from the city for their cure. The doctor related how another well-known professor in Moscow also sent most of his patients to live in a village during treatment. What is the great evil existing in large cities? In a casual conversation with the author, an outstanding San Francisco physician stated it in this one significant sentence: 'More than 75% of the diseases contracted by our patients are due to our drinking water which flows through hundreds of miles of pipes before it reaches the kitchen.'

"Frankly, the verdict of this prominent physician is rather severe, yet there is more truth than poetry in it. Piped water is a demon destroying human health in our great American cities, working hand in hand with other little demons, such as canned food (especially in tin), cold-storage meat, bread in waxed cellophane wrappings that has been improperly baked, fat substitutes, lack of fresh air, carbon monoxide from gas engine exhausts, the nerve-wracking noise of street cars and factories , and the general high tension under city living conditions.

"Millions of people think that city water, traveling through miles of pipes, is the cheapest and most healthful water to be had... yet quite the opposite is true. In fact, the city dweller often pays 15 to 20 years of his life for the use of piped water... The writer insists that water flowing through pipes for hundreds of miles is suitable only for laundering, dishwashing and other domestic purposes; it should not be used for drinking or cooking.

"Of course, large pieces of metal are not found in piped water, but there are always minute particles which work more slowly but as harmfully. Have you ever observed an old water main that is being replaced? It is 'worn out' on both sides; the earth has eaten it away on the outside, the water on the inside. It stands to reason that those who drank the water slowly consumed the metal that had been worn away on the inside of the pipe. On all metal pipes there is a quantity of rust, visible and invisible. This is drawn with the water from the faucet; and, when drunk, passes into the intestinal tract from where it is eliminated with great difficulty. Usually it lodges somewhere and starts to work its way out by a short cut."

Chronic Poisoning From Metallic Tooth Fillings

If water flowing through metal pipes takes up metallic substances from the pipes, and is therefore harmful to health, what about metals dissolved from tooth fillings that are in constant contact with the saliva twenty-four hours a day and 365 days in the year? Acids in the mouth fluids should act on these fillings and cause a certain amount to be dissolved and to pass into the system. Often they give off a distinct metallic taste, which is especially noticeable after acid fruits or other acid foods are eaten, under which conditions a greater amount of metal is dissolved and taken up by the saliva. In most cases, however, even though they may give off a metallic taste, since they are in the mouth continually, one loses sensitivity to their taste. To prove this point, put a copper penny in one's mouth and one will immediately notice a copper taste, which results from a minute amount of copper being dissolved from the penny and reaching the taste buds of the tongue. However, if one had copper in one's mouth continually, in the form of copper tooth fillings, one would lose sensitivity to their taste, as in the case of other tooth fillings.

There is considerable scientific evidence that amalgam fillings are harmful. One of the first to point out this fact was Melville Keith, M.D., of Bellville, Ohio, who claimed that such fillings give off mercury, a poison, which, by affecting the auditory nerves, may cause deafness. Dr. Keith also pointed out that red-colored dentures also contain mercury, leading to similar harmful effects. He found that these disappeared when amalgam fillings were removed and red dentures were abandoned. He recommended the removal of all amalgam fillings and the replacement of colored dentures by uncolored ones.

Dr. Kieferle of San Diego also violently objected to the use of amalgam fillings, claiming that they are made of mercury, a soft metal which tends to find its way into the general circulation and cause chronic poisoning. He pointed out that contact of salt with mercury forms bichloride of mercury, a deadly poison. He recommended the removal of all amalgam fillings from the teeth, especially in cases where the individual suffered from the ill effects of such fillings, causing mercurial poisoning.

Some years ago, the writer has read in the *Journal of the American Medical Association* a report on blood tests made soon after the installation of an amalgam filling in the tooth of a patient, with the result that considerable mercury appeared in the blood. This would indicate that amalgam fillings may cause chronic mercurial poisoning, which, though unnoticed, may nevertheless be harmful. The experience of the writer and his friends has shown that the removal of amalgam tooth fillings, as well as the removal of all metal from the mouth, including gold inlays, crowns, etc., led to a definite improvement in health, marked especially by a calmer nervous system and the absence of the irritability that occurred previously, when metallic substances dissolved from fillings were continually irritating the nervous system.

Aside from an undesirable chemical effect of amalgam and other metallic fillings (and all metals dissolve, even though gold and platinum are harder and less soluble than the softer metals) is an equally undesirable electrical one. A dental expert has informed the writer that he has evidence that when both amalgam and gold fillings are in the mouth at the same time, their different electromotive potentials cause them to act like two poles of a battery and to form an electric circuit. Also, since it is known that the brain is an electrical apparatus through which currents of electricity are constantly flowing, would not the presence of metal in the mouth produce "static" or some sort of interference or disturbing effect on these electrical currents. That this is so is indicating by the calming influence which follows the removal of all metal fillings from the mouth.

According to the modern theory that teeth decay from within, rather than as a result of external bacterial attack, the removal of metal fillings from the teeth should not be objected to; for even if the cavity was left open (as occurred in several cases known to the writer), this would be less harmful than retaining undesirable metals in one's mouth. (However, metal fillings can be advantageously replaced by porcelein ones. As for plastic fillings and dentures, these are not advisable, since they tend to give off formaldehyde or other poisonous substances, especially on contact with hot food. The writer knows a case where a bad skin condition persisted so long as plastic dentures were worn, but ceased when they were replaced by rubber ones. However, one should avoid red rubber plates, whose red color is due to the presence of mercury, preferring uncolored amber ones.)

After telling several friends about the good effects of the removal of all metal from his mouth (including both amalgam fillings and gold inlays), they did the same, with uniformly excellent results. In many of these cases, removal of the fillings and inlays revealed the existence of decay underneath; and since the toxic products of such decay were denied an outlet, they affected the roots of the teeth, which became rotten and full of pus. Especially when the nerve of the tooth was killed by the dentist at the time the filling or inlay was put in, with the result that the tooth was dead, was there greatest likelihood for decay and bad roots to be found in such teeth. The question now arises: Which is better, to retain metal fillings with decay and rotten roots underneath, or to remove the fillings and so permit the products of such decay to find an exit, rather than be trapped there, becoming increasingly toxic? Surely the removal of the filling, under such conditions is preferable. Dentists often notice upon removal of a crown that highly offensive odors are given off, due to decomposition products that were trapped by the crown, under which tooth decay has been going on.

According to the newer conception that teeth decay from within, rather due to bacterial attack from without, it is clear that plugging teeth with metal does not stop decay, which will proceed under the fillings, so long as the nutritional causes of tooth decay are not eliminated. Under such conditions, the fillings do more harm than good, since they prevent the products of decay, which goes on underneath them, to be trapped and denied an exit, whereupon they become highly toxic and are reabsorbed into the blood-stream. On the other hand, when the cavity is open, these highly toxic products can escape. There is some evidence that when the diet is properly balanced, tooth decay will stop, and that open cavities can do no harm. In some exceptional cases they have been known to fill in by themselves, or at least to become covered with a protective coating of enamel.

The writer knew a young lady who, though living on a very careful diet, suffered from persistent, and apparently incurable, stomach distress. All food disagreed with her. Her only remedy for her troubles was to abstain from food altogether, which she did for days at a time. The condition made her very moody and despondent, and produced undesirable psychic effects. She was, however, able to take liquids without difficulty, but not solid foods that required chewing. Eating a whole orange produced distress, but orange juice did not.

Examining her mouth, it was found that practically every tooth was filled with a large amalgam filling or inlay, since she was not financially able to afford gold. The writer concluded that she was suffering from chronic mercury poisoning, which metal she swallowed with every morsel of food she chewed; and that it was the mercury that she ingested with her food that caused everything she ate to disagree. The writer explained to her his analysis of her case and recommended the removal of the amalgam fillings and their replacement by porcelein ones. This was done, leading to a remarkable improvement in her health and well-being, physically and mentally. She developed a wonderful appetite; and all foods she ate now agreed with her. Her former moods and despondency disappeared; and her nervous system became more stable. It was noticed that underneath the amalgam fillings that were removed, decay existed, and a horrible putrid odor was given off. Absorption into the blood-stream of these decomposition products resulting from decay underneath her fillings must have contributed to her previous poor health and irritable nervous system, both of which conditions were remedied by the removal of the fillings. The writer suggested the replacement of amalgam fillings by porcelein ones only because he knew the young lady would object to having open cavities in her mouth, though it cannot be denied that open cavities are much goes on and decomposition products are trapped and absorbed into the blood-stream, to poison the entire body.

Aluminum Contamination of City Water

The anti-fluoridationists give us the impression that once the fluoridation of city water does not occur, such water is fit to drink, which is not the case at all, since fluorine is only one among many other poisons now added to city water supplies. It is merely one tenacle of the octopus of water contamination, which is ruining the health of the American people. Another tenacle is chlorination; and another is aluminization, or addition of aluminum compounds to water supplies for disinfecting purposes, as well as for filtration.

Sale of aluminum compounds to the water departments of big cities yields immense profits to the aluminum trust, just as does the sale of its by-product, sodium fluoride, for fluoridation purposes. This trust is behind the propaganda in favor of fluoridation, though in the case of the addition of aluminum to city water, since this is a universal practice and since no opposition to it has arisen, no propaganda campaign is necessary. Nor could such a campaign be possible, since, while in the case of fluorine, it is claimed to benefit the enamel of the teeth, in the case of aluminum, it is known to be a poison and to have no physiological function.

As an example of the present contamination of city water supplies with aluminum and other harmful chemicals, the city of Columbus, Ohio, each year, adds the following quantities of poisonous chemicals to its water: 500 tons of bauxite (aluminum ore), 8,000 tons of lime, 3,000 tons of soda ash, 1,200 tons of sulphuric acid, 500 tons of coke and 8 tons of liquid chlorine. Fort Lauderdale, Florida, adds to its water supply 40,000 tons of alum (aluminum) within a period of three months, or one pound per capita per month.

Aluminum sulphate is widely used for purposes of water filtration. In place of the older and safer method of "Slow Sand Filtration", formerly employed, the aluminum interests succeeded in introducing the new "Quick Sand Filtration" method, involving the addition of aluminum compounds to our drinking water. The impurities that were removed by this new method of filtration were much less harmful than the substance added to water to remove them - aluminum, a poisonous metal which remains in the water so filtered. This practice has brought huge profits to the aluminum trust, as well as many new serious chronic degenerative diseases to the American people, chief among which is cancer. On this subject, Dr. W.E.Holder, a Canadian scientist who has devoted many years to the study of the chemical contamination of drinking water, in his book, "Why Humanity Suffers", writes:

"A few years ago, it is presumed, vested interests, in order to get rid of their product, suggested the use of a coarser sand and in using aluminum sulphate (which is a salt of aluminum which has been boiled with sulphuric acid), which is soluble in water and is used as a mordant in dyeing, waterproofing cloth, sizing of paper and a most effective embalming fluid. By drinking plenty of this water we are slowly under the process of embalming.

"Chemical interests pointed out that if a coarser sand was used, with the addition of aluminum sulphate, a gelatinous film would be formed on the coarse grains of sand, and this would detain the bacteria and prevent them from passing through the filter. <u>But they did not state that the aluminum sulphate would not be destroyed but would pass through the filter.</u>

"It is stated that only one part is used to 70,000 parts of water. This is most interesting and may be all right in a way, but what must be the cumulative effect when all food is cooked in such water as well as being used for drinking? The aluminum sulphate passes out with the water through the filter and does not consume itself.

"It is suggested that aluminum sulphate destroys bacteria. If it does, why does chlorine have to be used in conjunction with it? Aluminum sulphate will clarify - make water clearer, the same as it does to beer and wine - but outside of that there is no benefit to the water.

"The composition of aluminum sulphate is worth a little study. It is prepared by boiling aluminum with sulphuric acid so that it becomes soluble in water. We know sulphuric acid is escharotic - it burns. We also know that aluminum coming in contact with other substances is also escharotic. We also know that one tablespoonful or less of sulphuric acid or two ounces of aluminum sulphate, either administered in a single dose, is sufficient to cause death.

"I have stated and have never been contradicted that aluminum sulphate is the cause of cancer and many other diseases...We have to remember that we have been taking this aluminum sulphate into the body for many years, even from infancy; the cells of the body are saturated with it. We can record it on our metallic recording machine; therefore this is no guesswork.

"At the present time, and for many years past, the question is: Why have the health and medical authorities allowed aluminum sulphate to be used in water filtration? Are they ignorant of its danger? Personally, I can hardly reconcile myself to this.

"Of course it is a good paying proposition for chemical manufacturers. I have before me a record from a city in the U.S.A. which has a high cancer rate, high percentage of sickness and a high death rate. In 1926 the expenditure of $55,000.00 was allotted to purchase 2,200 tons of aluminum sulphate for their water division. 'Nice pickings'. Then we have many other interests, such as pharmaceutical interests which benefit from the ill-health of the people. And lastly, organized medicine, hospitalization and eventually morticians. "

Dr. Holder claims that cities which employed the old-fashioned "slow sand filtration" method, which consisted in allowing water to pass through a bed of fine sand, as was the practice a half a century ago, had less epidemics and a lower death rate than occurs today in cities where the "quick sand filtration" method, involving the addition of aluminum compounds to water, is employed. The replacement of the older by the newer method, with the coincident addition of aluminum to drinking water, was accompanied by a marked increase in incidence of cancer, which Dr. Holder considers to be due to chronic aluminum poisoning - from drinking water, use of aluminum cooking utensils, use of chemical fertilizers, which cause plants to take up large amounts of aluminum from the soil, which they otherwise would not do, etc. Concerning the harmful effect of addition of aluminum to our drinking water , J.I.Rodale, in an article, "Shall Aluminum Utensils be Used in Cooking? " , in the April 1953 issue of Prevention, says:

"Alum is used in practically every city water works to kill certain bacteria in it. Alum is very high in aluminum, which is how it gets its name. On certain days, when the alum is placed in the water, its content may be very high, becoming gradually dissipated as the days go on. Should a group meal containing potato salad or sauerkraut (prepared and stored in an aluminum container) take place on a day when the city water has been given the benefit of a shot of alum, trouble might ensue.

"This reminds me of a fact related to me years ago by a man who runs a fish market. In his place of business most of his fish are dead, but he keeps some alive for particular customers. He told me that on the day when the city water receives its charge of chlorine, his fish die. The lesson here would be to attempt to work out a method where smaller amounts of these chemicals are applied every day, rather than in larger weekly or monthly doses. Of course the most valuable lesson would be to attempt to discover safer methods to purify our city waters, and do away with chlorine and alum as disinfectants. (You know that any disinfectant is bound to be a poison.)

In a work,"The Clinical Aspect of Chronic Poisoning by Aluminum and Its Alloys" by Leo Spira, M.D., with a foreword by Prof. Hans H. Meyer of the University of Vienna, cases are cited of severe skin conditions, accompanied by gastro-intestinal symptoms, which refused to clear up until the use of aluminum cooking utensils and 'aluminized or chlorinated tap water' was discontinued. Dr. Spira says:"A complete cure, not obtainable by any other means of treatment applied hitherto, was maintained as long as the patients persevered with the regime prescribed to them. They were put gradually on a regular diet but were not allowed to use aluminum utensils, tap water or any other source of metallic contamination...The symptom-complex described is caused by one or several irritants contained in aluminum utensils and in chlorinated or aluminized tap water."

Dr. Holder has done a valuable work in revealing the grave danger that lurks in the aluminizing of our drinking water, which he found to be a universal practice and which he considers to be an important cause of cancer. He says: "Organized medicine and other associates cannot any longer hide the true facts as to the danger that lurks in drinking water supplied to the public as being pure and fit for human consumption, when in fact the water supplied in most cities is an absolute danger to the community, and is the bearer of many diseses which are supposed to be mysterious and obscure."

Is Aluminum Poisoning Responsible for the Modern Increase of Nervous and Mental Diseases?

That aluminum is a poisonous metal which serves no physiological function, and which, when ingested, acts as a poison, tending to cause serious chronic degenerative diseases, such as cancer, has been suspected by a number of modern scientists. Dr. Charles Betts, who has studied this problem for over a quarter of a century, in his book, "Aluminum Poisoning", presents the scientific evidence in favor of the view that aluminum, dissolved from cooking utensils and derived from other sources (alum-containing baking powder, etc.), is a cause of cancer, ulcers, and nervous and mental diseases. Dr. Holder shares the same view, and considers city drinking water partly responsible for widespread aluminum poisoning, not to mention the use of chemical fertilizers. Keens, an English soil scientist, has shown that chemical fertilizers tend to make otherwise insoluble aluminum compounds in the soil abnormally soluble, so that plants take up an excess of metallic aluminum, which they communicate to consumers. This fact has been experimentally demonstrated by Dr. Holder by analysis of the aluminum content of chemically fertilized vegetables as compared with those grown naturally. When such vegetables are cooked in aluminum cooking utensils, together with aluminized tap water, their aluminum content, and cancer-producing capacity, is further increased. Testing most foods and beverages people use, Dr. Holder found that they are all very high in aluminum content. "How is it possible to combat disease", he asks, "when the people are supplied with contaminated water, which has a cumulative effect?

Concerning the harmful effects of small amounts of aluminum, ingested in the form of foods cooked in aluminum cooking utensils, water treated with aluminum compounds and foods grown with chemical fertilizers, the U.S. Dispensatory (1928) issues the following warning:

"When small quantities of the soluble salts of aluminum are introduced into the circulation, they produce a slow poisoning characterized by motor palsies and areas of local anesthesia, with fatty degeneration of the kidneys and liver; there are also symptoms of gastro-intestinal inflammation which is presumably the result of the effort of the glands of the intestinal tract to eliminate the poisoning."

In Report No. 78 of the British Ministry of Health we read the following concerning the injurious cumulative effects of continued intake of small quantities of aluminum:

"It is conceivable that extremely small amounts of aluminum, gaining access to the blood, might immobilize or affect adversely some consistuents which operate normally in resisting disease."

The U.S.A. Materia Medica, Therapeutics and Pharmacology says: "Aluminum hydroxide - this agent produces profound prostration with irritation of the mucous membrane with diminished secretions and as a result there is inactivity of the bowels. The nervous system is affected, as is indicated by the extreme prostration with numbness of the parts and paralysis of the involuntary muscles."

Dr. Holder's researches have shown that daily ingestion of aluminum compounds in drinking water is especially injurious to the nervous system; and for this reason he considers aluminum poisoning from drinking water as a cause of polio, as well as various nervous and mental diseases. It has been shown that ingested aluminum is stored principally in the brain and spinal cord, as well as in the liver, kidneys, spleen and thyroid.

An important reason why aluminum compounds profoundly affect the nervous system is because they tend to disturb phosphorus metabolism, causing phosphorus to be eliminated in the feces, when it otherwise would function as part of brain and nerve tissue. A large percentage of phosphorus becomes insoluble by combination with aluminum; and since phosphorus is an essential component of all cellular nuclei, where it is present in the form of lecithin, it is clear that by its tendency to make phosphorus unavailable to the organism and by preventing the formation of lecithin, aluminum leads to a phosphorus-lecithin deficiency which profoundly affects the central nervous system. By depriving the nerve and brain cells of lecithin, it produces despondency, anxiety, phobia and other abnormal psychoneurotic conditions.

That the modern practices of aluminizing drinking water, cooking in aluminum utensils and chemical fertilization of the soil have a relation to the recent terrific increase in nervous and mental diseases there can be no doubt. The writer has heard of a case of insanity diagnosed as due to aluminum brain poisoning; and he believes that there exist many more such cases incorrectly diagnosed as to their real origin. For there can be no doubt that due to its capacity to withdraw lecithin from the brain and nervous system, aluminum can profoundly affect the functioning of both. Studies have shown that while the normal brain contains about 28% lecithin, the brains of the insane contain about 14%, or half as much. An eminent German biochemist has coined the phrase, "Ohne phosphor keinen gedenken" (without phosphorus, no thought) - so that it is clear that by its tendency to rob lecithin from the spinal cord and brain, aluminum may be a cause of polio and other nervous diseases.

Commenting on the treatment of aluminum-caused neurological and psychiatric conditions, Schmidt and Hoagland of the United States Department of Agriculture write :

"Phosphorus is widely distributed in the body as an essential component of every cell. It is important in the formation of phosphorized fat, called lecithin. This is a dominant factor in nerve function.

"A disturbance of their normal relationship as by a phosphorus deficiency is of vital consequence...As a treatment, all the remedies in any therapy will avail nothing if aluminum is not excluded. A disease syndrome may be removed, but by the undermining, insidious action of the aluminum and its alloys, the general march of destruction will continue."

Dr. Holder comments: "The above gives us a pretty good inkling as to the cause of many mental cases, especially in middle life. Then again, we must not lose sight of the fact that as we increase in age, even if the intake of aluminum is of infinitely small quantity, we obtain the cumulative effects, no matter from what source they may be derived."

Dr. Holder cites the following two cases of aluminum poisoning reported by two medical men. The first report comes from Dr. Stearns:

"One case that I saw in consultation, who was in extremis and died within a few days, gave a high degree of aluminum poisoning. She had a fulminating cancer of the pharynx."

The second case was reported by Dr. Heimbach:

"I am very anxious to enumerate a few experiences I have had with aluminum poisoning. Two acute cases very nearly died; in fact, one did die from a stroke. The other, a very close friend of mine, a veteran of World War I, was taken with severe abdominal pains and vomiting and diarrhea at first. In a day or two it reverted into constipation and we couldn't get anything through at all. The pain was so intense for a while that I feared it may be a surgical case. I couldn't convince myself that it was appendicitis, but I soon discovered it was aluminum poisoning. He made a complete recovery and has been well since.

"Another peculiar case puzzled me for quite a while. She had an ulcer of the leg, probably four or five inches in diameter. She responded to treatment and the ulcer healed up, but by the time the ulcer healed up she began to get necrosis over the abdomen and that started to necrose across. Then she got acute obstruction of the intestines and died in a very short time. A portion of the liver and some of the tissues over the abdomen were sent to a chemist who had become interested in the question. He made a test and the report came back that there was aluminum in all the tissues which had been sent to him."

Aluminized City Water, Pasteurized Milk and Insecticide Residues in Foods as Causes of Polio

We have shown above that the water supplied to the inhabitants of American cities is poisoned by chemicals and metals, including chlorine and aluminum. Dr. Holder claims that aluminum is a cumulative poison which, taken into the system in the form of drinking water, may settle in the spinal cord; and that polio may be a result of such poisoning affecting the sensitive organism of the child. He considers use of pasteurized milk and vegetables and fruits containing toxic spray residues as other possible causes.

Dr. Holder's tests have shown that pasteurized milk has a surprising high metallic content; and he considers this metallic content of pasteurized milk as a cause of polio. It appears that during the pasteurization process the milk becomes contaminated with metals, probably as the result of being heated in metallic containers.

On the subject of insecticide residues in foods as possible causes of polio, we quote from an article, "Many Prevalent Diseases Blamed on Insecticides" by John P. Plum, writing in the Times-Herald of Washington, D.C. some years ago:

"Many stomach, intestinal and other ills of today, including some that resemble polio, may be caused by deadly insecticides used in the growing of fruit and vegetable crops, authorities in both medicine and pharmacology admitted last night.

"This startling disclosure came as the Food and Drug Administration prepared to begin extensive hearings Jan. 17 into amounts of 'poisonous or deleterious' residues carried by many fruits and vegetables sent to market.

"Dr. Paul B. Dunbar, commissioner, said toxicologists are 'worried about chronic poisoning resulting from the long-time consumption of minute amounts of a poison which may eventually build up in the system to produce a serious physical disturbance.'

"Dr. Abraham Gelperin, director, Bureau of Communicable Diseases and Assistant Clinical Professor of Public Health at Yale University, stated flatly that he believes many ills are the result of such poisoning.

"Both Dunbar and Gelperin pointed out that arsenic and lead have cumulative effects and that there is much to be learned about a few of the newer insecticides.

"Among the newer group are the organic phosphate type developed in this country since the war. One of these is parathion, now used commercially on a large scale throughout the nation.

"One of its manufacturers describes it as capable of producing severe toxic effects and death in animals and man, either by oral administration, inhalation of mists, dusts or vapors, and by absorption through the unbroken skin.

"Dr. Arnold J. Lehman, Chief, Division of Pharmacology, Food and Drug Administration, stated the organic phosphates are three to five times as toxic as nicotine and that 12 milligrams or one third of a grain of parathion or tetraethyl pyrophosphate may be considered as a poisonous quantity and liable to prove fatal.

"Dr. J.G. Townsend, medical director, U.S. Public Health Industrial Hygiene Division, said one of its symptoms is 'extreme muscular weakness' and that it is possible that some sickness mistaken for polio may have been caused by eating fruits or vegetables bearing parathion residue.

"Far Stronger than DDT

"He described the newer phosphate insecticides as far more virulent than anything ever used before in agricultural pest control.

"It would be 'pretty tough' on people if produce or fruit sprayed or dusted with dilute forms recommended by manufacturers reached market before ample time was allowed for the residue to disappear, Townsend stated.

"Some medical authorities see more than a coincidence in the distribution and use of parathion for the first time in 1948 and the epidemics of polio in sections of the country last year.

"Symptoms of parathion poisoning are similar to those of polio, including headache, gastric upset, giddiness, tightness of the chest, vomiting and sometimes diarrhea.

"Gelperin said he thinks large numbers of what are believed to be polio cases are in reality poisoning cases, possibly caused by something like parathion.

"Parathion and related insecticides are too new to know what effects their use on crops might have on consumers of those crops over an extended period."

It is claimed that profound calcium deficiency is a cause of polio. Since the pasteurization process renders most of the calcium of milk unavailable, pasteurized milk has been considered a cause of polio for this reason. Likewise the phosphoric acid present in soft drinks, by its tendency to withdraw calcium from the system, has also been considered a cause of polio among children who are large consumers of such beverages.

The Origin of Cancer

The origin of cancer now baffles medical science. Dr. Holder, in two works he has published on this subject, traces this disease to two main causes: (1) cholesterol derived from use of dairy products, and (2) metallic poisoning by aluminum in foods and water, due to use of chemical fertilizers, addition of aluminum compounds to city water, use of aluminum cooking utensils, etc.

Dr. Holder claims that there is a marked difference between animal cholesterol, as present in cow's milk, cream, butter and cheese, and human cholesterol, which is a prime constituent of the brain and nervous system, as well as of all cells of the body. He claims that the intermixing of both types of cholesterol causes a colloidal degeneration in the cells, which leads to the development of cancer. Also, foods grown with chemical fertilizers, he believes, change the manner in which cholesterol functions in the body and encourage its deposit in the form of cancerous growths. But it is especially the excessive intake of foreign animal cholesterol, by the use of milk, butter, cheese and lard which he considers to be a fundamental cause of cancer. (All animal foods are rich in cholesterol, and therefore cancer-producing.)

Hand in hand with increased consumption of cholesterol-containing foods in modern times has been the increased intake of aluminum in the form of drinking water, foods cooked in aluminum pots and the use of chemical fertilizers, all of which are considered partly responsible for the modern increase of cancer. The relation between intake of cholesterol and aluminum, and incidence of cancer, is shown by the following table prepared by Dr. Holder, based on one drawn up by Keens, based on statistics furnished by the British Health Department:

COMPARISON OF TH INCREASED USE OF DAIRY PRODUCTS AND ALUMINUM POISONING FROM TOXIC SOILS IN RELATION TO THE SPREAD OF CANCEROUS DISEASES OF PLANTS, ANIMALS AND HUMANS

Year		Per million per year Human Deaths From Cancer
1842	Natural manure used exclusively for fertilizing. Chemical fertilizers were unknown. Very little milk used.	173
1843-50	Chemical fertilizers first introduced. Propaganda for increased use of milk commenced and more milk consumed	274
1890	Chemical fertilizers used on more widespread scale and increased consumption of milk	701
1900	Still more chemical fertilizers used and milk consumption greatly increased	1,001

Year		Per million per year Deaths from Cancer
1912	Food and mouth disease of animals caused by chemically formed virus (chemical fertilizers)	1,019
1917	57% of cattle suffer from bovine tuberculosis. Still greater consumption of milk. Cancer discovered in field mice and other animals	1.192
1922	New root rot of vegetables caused by supposed parasitic fungi (really caused by chemical fertilizers). Intense propaganda to increase sale of milk.	1.229
1927	Milk consumption increased 40%. Aluminum cooking utensils introduced	1,376
1932	Large quantities of potatoes lost as result of new disease. 3,000,000 acres of land taken out of use as unfit for cultivation due to having been ruined by chemical fertilizers. Consumption of milk again increased	1,510
1936	Rampant diseases of crops, cattle, sheep, humans	1,563

The Menace of Fluoridation

In an article, "Poison on Tap", in the January 1954 issue of <u>Organic Gardening and Farming</u>, M.C.Goldman writes:

"The Age of Chemicals races haphazardly on -- and every consumer of food and water becomes an increasing loser in that race. In the food realm, skyrocketing chemicalization has ordained a saturation of our land with life-and-fertility draining synthetic fertilizers, and of our foodstuffs with appallingly toxic insecticides, fungicides, herbicides, preservatives, color and flavor additives, spoilage retarders - and who-knows-what-next! ... Now we are huzzahed and 'modernistically' stampeded into sanctioning an even more direct poisoning - the very scientific dumping of fluorine - an admittedly potent element, an actual rat killer - into our public water supplies.

"The strongest argument against any hasty approval of putting even small doses of the rat poison in anyone's drinking water is the fact that there is no safe assurance of what the accumulated added fluorine will do to vital body organs, blood, bones and yes, even teeth, oever a period of years. On the contrary, there is mounting evidence - increasing actual experiments and survey reports - which indicates that many of the definite hazards involved in water fluoridation far outweigh the solitary, limited, <u>possible</u> benefit it might

This "benefit" is the claim that since fluorine is a constituent of the tooth enamel, and since this mineral tends to be lacking in most diets, its addition to drinking water should harden and strengthen the enamel and so reduce the incidence of dental cavities! However, those who advocate water fluoridation for this reason fail to realize that while <u>organic</u> fluorine compounds, as present in foods grown on the fluorine-rich soil of Deaf Smith County, Texas, where there is a remarkable absence of tooth decay, may be utilized by the body and build stronger teeth, <u>inorganic</u> fluorine compounds, as provided by the sodium fluoride added to drinking water, cannot be readily utilized by the body, which is unable to assimilate minerals in inorganic form. Such inorganic minerals are not only valueless, but harmful. Proof of this is afforded by the fact that in regions where drinking water is naturally high in inorganic fluorine compounds they tend to cause mottling of teeth. Since sodium fluoride, added to drinking water in cities where fluoridation is practiced, is an inorganic compound of fluorine, its action on the teeth, like that of other inorganic fluorides, must be injurious, rather than beneficial.

Sodium fluoride is so virulent a poison that if it comes in contact with the feet or legs of rats, death may result. Non-fatal doses of fluorides can cause cachexia, as in cancer and tuberculosis. Even in minute quantities, as present in fluoridated water, sodium fluoride is harmful. Its use by pregnant mothers is considered a cause of fatalities due to premature birth. It is also considered to cause sterility, or at least to predispose to this condition. Damage to the brain and nerve cells has been reported to result from the use of such water. What will kill a rat in high concentration should prove injurious to a human being in small concentration, especially if its intake continues day after day over a period of years. It is well known that sodium fluoride is a cumulative poison.

"An excess of fluorides in drinking water has mottled the teeth in various American communities. Who will guarantee that if fluoride is diluted one part to a million of water, as advocated, that it may not have some prolonged, insidious effect?" So writes George A. Swandiman, D.D.S., of Grand Forks, S.D., in an article, "The Argument Against Fluoridating City Water". He writes: "Fluorides are extremely corrosive and are used for etching glass. Fluorides also are used as a highly potent rat poison. I do not crave rat poison, even well diluted. How do I know that this poison will not have a cumulative effect? Suppose this diluted rat poison gradually ruins my kidneys and thus sends me to my grave. Will it be any comfort to me if my dental association says, 'He died with perfect teeth.' As an American citizen, I crave to be treated neither as a rat nor a guinea pig."

Sodium fluoride is a by-product of the aluminum industry, which has found big profit in selling it to the water departments of cities for the fluoridation of water. This otherwise unsaleable aluminum waste, when once dumped into the Gulf of Mexico, killed all fish for miles around and poisoned the Gulf feed-beds for two years. Yet it is now being added to the water that the American people drink, and in more and more cities.

The chemical contamination of our drinking water by chlorine, aluminum and fluorine poses a real problem to the health-seeker who finds himself a victim of a world in which water as well as foods are systematically poisoned. The purest and best water is the water found in coconuts, but this is not always available and is expensive. The most practical solution of the problem is to secure a glass distilling apparatus and prepare one's own pure distilled water - much purer than commercial distilled water made in a metallic apparatus from which it often acquires a metallic taste.

Glass-distilled water Versus Commercial (Metal-Distilled) Water

In view of the chemical poisoning of city water supplies, Dr. Holder offers the following advice: "The only antidote to overcome the danger in using city tap water is to use distilled water...Only distilled water should be used for drinking in schools. Only distilled water should be used in factories. (I have received many adverse reports after the drinking of present tap water and milk.)"

7   There are two kinds of distilled water: (1) commercial distilled water, as used for storage batteries, which is produced in a metallic distilling apparatus, and (2) glass-distilled water, as made by chemists in laboratories, who use a glass distilling apparatus for making water of optimal purity for delicate analytical work, purer than commercial distilled water.

Dr. Holder formerly accepted the common belief that all distilled water was pure H_2O. However, much to his surprise, he discovered that commercial distilled water (produced by the action of hot steam against cooled walls of metallic condensing tubes) did contain a certain amount of metallic substances, though less than present in tap water. For this reason water distilled in a glass apparatus is best, since there is no possibility of it picking up metals dissolved from the condensing tubes in which it is made.

If foods cooked in metal pots, whether aluminum, iron or stainless steel, dissolve and take up metal dissolved from their walls, so distilled water takes up metal from the apparatus in which it is formed; and just as glass cooking utensils are safest to use, than glass distilling apparatus will produce purer distilled water than a metallic one. Dr. Holder writes:

"I have a chemist come in to do my analytical work. A short time ago I had been making some experiments in sterilizing milk by an electrical process, and we decided to see if culture would develop in water which had undergone treatment by electrical process... We tested out the tap water first and found it showed 35 units of metallic. My chemist said he would not use the tap water, but would use distilled water, which he knew would be all right. However, I decided to test the distilled water, to the amazement of the chemist and myself, it showed seven units of metallic.

The chemist was astounded, for he had always understood distilled water was free from contamination. I asked him what effect this would have on medicine prescriptions 'aqua pura' in addition to drugs. He stated that although the amount may be small, it certainly would have a great bearing on the action of the drugs prescribed."

The distilled water to which Dr. Holder here refers is commercial distilled water, whose metallic taste evidently is due to its metallic content, derived from the metallic apparatus in which it is produced. For maximum purity, a glass distilling apparatus should be used. Recently the writer has perfected such an apparatus for producing a home supply of pure distilled water for kitchen use. It is known as the "Home Distilling Apparatus" and is for sale by Organic Food Research Associates, 215 Sixth Street, Lorain, Ohio.

The writer has himself used glass-distilled water exclusively for some twenty years, with excellent results. A friend of his, who also used only glass-distilled water which he made in his own distillator, once questioned the head of a water company manufacturing absolutely pure and equal to glass-distilled water. The latter replied that he could not honestly answer this question in the affirmative.

Water is often triple-distilled, since the first distilling does not completely eliminate all the impurities, especially those that are volatile and which pass up in the steam and reappear in the distilled water. Since both chlorine and fluorine are volatile substances the question arises, when city water is distilled, whether some chlorine and fluorine may not pass into the distilled water. It is best, if possible, to start the distillation process with the purest possible water, using spring water in preference to city water. Those who consider spring water as being pure and harmless will be surprised at the ugly-looking precipitate of calcium carbonate and other inorganic deposits that remain behind in the distilling flask, and which, when spring water is drunk, tend to settle along the inner walls of the arteries and in other parts of the body, hastening the advent of the ossifying processes that cause the symptoms of old age.

Is Spring Water Safe to Drink? Does It Calcareous Deposits?

Health reformers who denounce the chlorination and fluoridation of water, when asked what kind of water one should use, generally recommend spring water, giving the impression that is is absolutely pure and harmless. But is it really pure and harmless

Chemical analysis show that all spring water, whether hard or soft, contains a large quantity of inorganic minerals which the body cannot use, and which, since they cannot be assimilated or fulfill any physiological function (since the body can assimilate and use minerals only when in organic combination.), Must be harmful. It is for this reason that belief in the therapeutic value of mineral water, like the belief in the efficiency and value of drugs, is without scientific basis. The inorganic lime of spring water, rather than provide available calcium for building teeth, tends to settle in the joints and in other parts of the body as calcareous deposits, just as it coats the inner wall of a tea kettle.

While we consider it best to use spring water for distilling pruposes, if it is unavailable, we must admit that distilled city water is infinitely purer and better than city water which has not been distilled; and, under such conditions, should be used.

Were spring water obtained directly from springs, as obtained during camping trips, it would not be so bad, but commercial bottled spring water is the product of a bottling factory, and, as is true of bottled milk, must pass through bottling machinery for mass production. And as in the case of piped water, spring water must pass through pipes in being pumped up; and comes in contact with metal all the way from its source to the bottle, in the factory where it is bottled.

But even if spring water is secured directly from springs as in olden times, and does not come in contact with metal pipes, pumps and bottling machinery, it is not entirely pure, since it contains inorganic minerals which the body cannot use, and which are more or less harmful, tending to promote the formation of calcareous deposits in the organism. This is especially true when such water is hard. For a long time it was believed that goiter was caused by use of hard water, causing lime deposits in the thyroid gland, for which reason this disease is common in regions where water is exceptionally hard, as in parts of the Swiss Alps. Paracelsus held this view years ago; and Dr. Robert McCarrison, in his work on goiter, substantiates it, considering calcareous deposits in the thyroid as one among other causes of this disease.

About a century ago, an English chemist named Rowbatham claimed that use of ordinary spring water, as well as well water, due to its content of inorganic minerals which the body cannot use and which tend to form deposits, is a cause of the gradual ossification of the organism manifesting in the symptoms of senility. To avoid such calcareous deposits, he advised the use of distilled water. An English physician, Dr. De Lacy Evans, in his book, "How To Prolong Life", expressed the same view, and also recommended distilled water to preserve youth and ward off the ageing process which he considered hastened by use of ordinary water containing calcareous matter. Rowbatham writes:

"Spring water contains an amount of earthly ingredients which is fearful to contemplate. It certainly differs very much in different districts and at various depths, but it has been calculated that water of an average quality contains so much carbonate and other compounds of lime, that a person drinking an average amount each day will, in forty years, have taken into the body as much as would form a pillar of solid chalk or marble as large as a good-sized man. So great is the amount of lime in spring water, that the quantity taken daily would alone be enough to choke up the system, so as to bring on decrepitude and death long before we arrive at twenty years of age, were it not for the kidneys and other secreting organs throwing it off in considerable quantities."

However, with advancing years, the eliminating organs, as the kidneys and the pores of the skin, gradually become weakened and falter in their functions, so that a certain percentage of calcareous matter remains in the body and is not eliminated. It gradually accumulates in various tissues in the form of calcareous deposits, slowly changing the flexibility of youth into the rigidity of old age. If we observe how a tea kettle becomes plastered at the bottom and on the sides with incrustations of a hard, stony substance from the water boiled therein, then we shall have an idea of how the internal coat of the blood vessels and other organs become hardened by the incrustations of calcareous matter that gradually deposits in them as the organism commences to age.

Clear evidence of this fact is afforded by placing some spring water into the flask of a glass distilling apparatus and distilling it. One will then be surprised at the large quantity of calcium carbonate and other compounds of lime that remain behind and are clearly visible in the form of a white chalky deposit that lines the inner wall of the flask, and which must be removed at frequent intervals by a solution of hydrochloric acid. By distilling the spring water one avoids the intake of this calcareous matter which settles in the body just as it settles in the distilling flask. Since it is inorganic, the body cannot use it, as it can use organic compounds of lime. It is harmful and should be avoided. For this reason it is best to distill all spring water before using.

In his "Materia Medica", Dr. Thompson says that the inorganic lime compounds in spring water is the cause of gravel and calculus complaints which Dr. Percival and others have observed to be common in regions where hard water is drunk. Such observations have led several writers to conclude that hard water is an important contributing cause of the calcification processes that accompany premature old age, including hardening of the arteries. Concerning the fact that calcareous degeneration is an important factor in the causation of premature senility, Dr. de la Torre writes: "Hard spring water, as well as the water we drink in cities, is impregnated with these very earthly substances (carbonate of lime, etc.) which greatly contribute to the ossification of body tissues. "

Dr. De Lacy Evans points out, that distilled water, due to its capacity to dissolve and help remove inorganic mineral deposits in the body, is valuable to help eliminate them and so retard the process of senile ossification, which will help to preserve youth and extend the life-span; and he therefore recommends the exclusive use of distilled water as a beverage by those who wish to live long. As we have already pointed out, the purest distilled water is water prepared at home in a glass distilling apparatus, rather than commercial distilled water, made in a metallic distilling apparatus.

Let us now consider two unfounded charges that some have made against the use of distilled water. The first is the fact that it lacks minerals the body needs, present in ordinary water, and also that it may dissolve out and remove minerals from the body. In answer to this we will say that the minerals of ordinary water are <u>inorganic</u>, and therefore the body cannot use them; and, as pointed out, they are harmful. Secondly, the minerals that distilled water dissolves and removes from the body are the harmful <u>inorganic</u> deposits which cause disease and old age, but not colloidal physiological minerals of cellular cytoplasm. Among the first of the harmful inorganic substances that distilled water helps eliminate are accumulated metallic residues, since these are most highly soluble. Hence a distilled water regimen, or the exclusive use of distilled water for drinking and cooking purposes, is valuable for the prevention of cancer and other metal-caused diseases.

The next objection against the use of distilled water is that, since it is not aerated or exposed to sunshine, as freely flowing spring water is, it is "dead" and lacks the "life" of other water. In reply we may say that neither has well water nor spring water pumped up from the earth been exposed to sunshine, nor aerated, as water derived from overground sources has been. This objection may, however, be overcome by exposing distilled water to the sunshine before using (which can be highly recommended, in view of the claim made by certain writers that such sun-irradiated water is highly beneficial), and by aerating it by pouring it from pitcher to pitcher, so that it falls through the air as far as possible while being poured. (In irradiating water, be sure to expose it directly to the sun's rays, since ultra-violate rays will not pass through ordinary glass.

What about well water? While well water, especially when brought up by the old-fashioned method with a water bucket (rather than being pumped up through pipes which tend to rust), is better than city water, it is open to the same objection as spring water, namely that it contains considerable inorganic substances which the body cannot use and which are harmful. There is still another objection, which has been pointed out by Dr. Holder, namely that when the well exists on or near farmlands where chemical fertilizers and sprays were used, residues from such fertilizers and sprays, by subterraneous seepage, may find their way into the well water, just as obnoxious substances and bacteria from cesspools and toilets in the immediate vicinity of the well may do. Today, when most soils in cultivation have been poisoned with chemical fertilizers and sprays, inhabitants of rural areas are often no more able to secure pure, chemical-free water than city people. Therefore, they have as much reason to distill their well water before using - aside from the fact that even under the best conditions, well water contains inorganic matter which is harmful to the organism and should be removed before using.

As for rain water, while pure rain water, collected from a non-soluble surface (not from a metal roof) and in a wooden barrel, would be ideal, since it has been naturally aerated in falling and never heated as distilled water has been, where can pure rain water be obtained today? Certainly not in the contaminated atmosphere of cities or around cities. And even if one goes as far as possible from large cities, one is not safeguarded against the contamination of rain water by radioactive dust and clouds, now known to be carried by winds for thousands of miles. In an article, "Slow Poisons Working," in the December 1952 Prevention, Dr.E.J.Ryan says : "I am a bit skeptical about what may be happening to us with all these atomic fission products floating around in the atmosphere. An atom bomb set off in the deserts of New Mexico may not kill anyone outright and dramatically, but how about all the radioactive particles that are windblown on high and deposited all over the country? Surely , someone is going to protest and say that unless a Geiger instrument can count the presence of these radioactive particles there is no danger involved. No physicist am I, but I feebly remark that Geiger counter or not, I am a bit uneasy with the thought that all these atomic fission products are drifting around, dropping in the soil from which our food comes, in the water we drink, in the air we breathe. Again I wonder what the cumulative effects of these sublethal atomic bombardments may be on the nation's health. "

It is claimed that certain vegetables examined in Los Angeles markets were found to give reactions of radioactivity - probably due to the reason Dr. Ryan suggested.

Metallic Contamination of Foods and Beverages by Grinding and Juicing Machines, Eating Utensils, Etc.

We have mentioned already that foods cooked in metallic pots, irrespective of the nature of the metal of which they are composed - whether aluminum, iron, copper or stainless steel - dissolve and take up certain quantities of these metals during the process of cooking; and that such metals are injurious to health. While stainless steel is the least harmful of the metals mentioned, it is nevertheless not entirely desirable. It is best to cook in glass. But even in this case, it is best to select glassware that contains the least metallic admixture, preferring the baking type casseroles (which may be used for cooking, if placed over asbestos pads) to the top-of-stove ware which contains a greater amount of metallic admixture.

Regarding food grinding machines, even when a visible uglylooking black substance is not given off, as sometimes occurs, there is always some metallic contamination, especially where the grinding process occurs by friction of metal parts against each other. Where grains are ground by the use of metal burrs, these visibly wear away and require replacement as time goes on. Where does the metal so worn away go to except into the flour or meal?

Without doubt, glass-enclosed liquefiers are preferable to metallic grinding and juicing machines, since their action does not depend on friction of metal parts against each other; and so they have less tendency to metallically contaminate foods than do these other machines. However, there is some metallic contact and possibility of metallic contamination, even though less than in the case of juicing machines.

Even when grain mills have stone burrs, which do not contaminate flours and meals with metallic substances, as do steel rollers and metal burrs on grain mills, the flour and meal produced by such machines cannot compare in health value with those produced by the old-fashioned slow action of stone-grinding by water power, or the stone-grinding by hand, as practiced by Indians, since in these cases vitamins are not destroyed by heat as generated by more rapidly rotating machine-driven burrs.

Contact of hot food with metals leads to a certain quantity of metal to pass into solution and contaminate such foods; and this occurs not only when foods are cooked in metal pots, but also when soups and other hot foods are mixed with metal utensils during cooking or serving. For this reason cooks employ large wooden spoons and forks in preference to metal ones. The Chinese, for the same reason, prefer wooden eating utensils to metal ones, their reason being that contact of hot foods, especially soups, with metal utensils leads to a certain metallic contamination, affecting both the taste and quality of foods. Use of wooden eating utensils, however, is not confined to the Chinese, but is widely practiced by many races, such as the Turks, etc.; and this is not due to lack of metal utensils, but rather to recognition of the superiority of wooden ones, for preserving the purity and flavor of foods. (The writer, for many years, has preferred to eat with wooden utensils whenever possible, finding that foods taste much better when they are used.)

Even in the case of raw foods, there is some evidence that they are best when served and eaten with non-metallic utensils. An example of this is the well-known practice of expert salad makers, not to cut up salads with a metal knife, but rather to break up their leaves with the fingers. It is claimed that salads thus prepared without metallic contact have more flavor. That this may be due to the fact that their vitamins are thus retained (and, being electrical in nature, metallic contact might "short-circuit" them and dissipate them), is proven by certain experiments which showed that when fruits and vegetables are cut with a metal knife their content of certain vitamins, especially vitamin C, is lower than when cut with a plastic, glass or wooden knife. Of course, when there are metal fillings in the teeth, these should exercise a similar effect in reducing the vitamin value of foods, which fact is indicated by the superior flavor that foods acquire after such fillings are removed from the mouth.

It is best to avoid all metallic contact of foods. The writer has found that it is best to use plastic graters in preference to metal ones. The former tend to preserve the vitamins of foods to a greater extent than the latter, which, like metal knives, tend to diminish the vitamin content of grated raw vegetables ; and the same occurs when vegetables are passed through metal juicing machines. The writer found that when carrots are grated with a plastic grater and then squeezed by hand through a cheesecloth, the carrot juice is much superior in health value than when prepared by the use of a machine or even when a metal grater is used. The same applies to other juices. For many years the writer used plastic, glass or wooden knives for cutting acid fruits and vegetables, rather than use metal ones, which are to some extent acted on by acids, which fact is often noticeable to the sense of taste, as when tomatoes are sliced with a metal knife.

As for the claim that contact of foods with plastics is harmful, this is certainly true in the case of hot foods, which visibly affect plastics, often causing them to warp. This is why plastic dentures are harmful, since they come into contact with hot foods, leading to danger of formaldehyde poisoning . However, when plastics come into contact with cold foods, they do not seem to affect the food in any harmful way, and are less dangerous than metals, which tend to dissolve in contact with liquids or acids. Hardwood utensils are of course better than plastic ones.

We can learn much from the traditional dietetic wisdom of the Chinese, whose practice of eating with chopsticks is not a product of a foolish superstition, but based on recognition of the fact that metallic contact of food is undesirable. For the same reason the Chinese prefer porcelein tea kettles to metal ones; and when metal pans are used for Chinese cooking, the practice is to simmer them in oil, rather than to cook in water, since metals are less soluble in oil than in water. In this connection, the following quotation which the writer found among his nutritional notes is interesting:

"The Chinese cook stuck the end of an ivory chopstick into a small brown biscuit.

"'Taste, sir!', he said. The biscuit was warm, crisp and rich. It was light, nutritious - a biscuit, in a word, of peculiar excellence. 'This biscuit, sir, is made of flour of lentils', said the Chinaman. Lentils are considered the most nutritious of all foods of the earth. This one lentil biscuit is equal in nourishment to a pound and a half of roast beef.' He then took from a tin a little cake. 'Again, taste', he said. The little cake was rich and good. 'It is made , sir, of the flour of almonds,' said the cook. 'Fresh, sweet almonds ground into a white powder between two mill stones. Such a flour is a finer thing than your flour of wheat, oh?'

"Then he lifted a great lid and revealed some thirty to forty compartments, one filled with a pink flour, another with a yellow, a third with a brown one, a fourth with a white, a fifth with a pale green, etc. 'All these are Chinese flours of rice, of peanuts, of beans, of potatoes, of sweet potatoes, peas, coconuts, millet, bananas - in fact, sir, we make a flour out of everything but wheat, and therefore the coarse, dry, tasteless flour of wheat is useless to us.'" (See below reasons why wheat is an inferior grain, which is uric-acid-forming and decalcifying.)

Coconut Water: The Supreme Distilled Water

There can be no doubt of the fact that no other water can equal coconut water, or the water found inside the coconut, for purity and health value. Throughout the tropics coconut water is the favorite beverage and is considered to have remarkable therapeutic value, especially in bladder and kidney conditions, both of which organs it cleanses and reinvigorates. No distilling apparatus that man can contrive can equal the coconut palm, which draws up moisture from the soil and naturally distills it to make a delicious and nutritious beverage, often called coconut milk, because it contains in dilute concentration all the elements of the coconut meat - proteins, fats, sugars, minerals and vitamins - all in solution in the purest distilled water that exists.

Those who wish the very best will purchase heavy water-laden coconuts wholesale by the hundred and will use coconut water in place of any other water, which is a common practice in the tropics, where coconut water is often used both for drinking and cooking, especially in regions where the natural water supply is contaminated. There is no finer neverage. One can live on it exclusively for long periods of time ; and the coconut water regimen has proven to possess great therapeutic value, superior to fasting, since it keeps the bowels open by its aperient action, while stimulating the kidneys and bladder to eliminate impurities from the blood-stream.

Those who consider this an expensive luxury should bear in mind the many diseases and cost of medical services, as a result of using chemical- and metal-containing ordinary water - diseases whose true origin is seldom admitted and which are attributed to other causes. It is much more sensible to spend the same money otherwise spent on illness to purchase coconuts in wholesale amounts and to use their water exclusively in place of other water. And incidentally, the solid meat of the coconut may find many culinary uses. From it a milk may be made which is far more healthful than cholesterol-containing cow's milk, a butter which is more healthful than cholesterol-containing cow's butter, an oil which is more healthful than acid-forming vegetable oils, and a cream which provides an alkaline salad dressing and which may also be used in cooking and baking in place of other less digestible and inferior fats .

CHAPTER FOUR

The Chemical Contamination of Bread

In the article "Poison by the Plateful" in the March 1954 issue of
<u>Organic Gardening and Farming</u>, M. C. Goldman writes:

> "Bread has been termed the 'staff of life,' but in the form most
> of us eat this staple, it is piteously weakened stuff. More than
> ten million pounds a year of synthetic food emulsifiers, or softeners,
> are now being used in bread, baked goods and other foods, although
> the question of their safety for human consumption remains unsettled.
> The DElaney Committee ascertained that in 1949 two companies alone
> sold 10,000,000 pounds of chemicals to some 30,000 bakers for uses as
> substitutes for milk, butter, eggs, essential oils and other materials.
> These replacements are nutritionally worthless, and the Committee's
> investigation found that bakers who had not adopted these polyoxythen
> type softeners used 41 per cent more natural shortening and 38 per
> cent more milk solids than those who had. Furthermore, the bleaching,
> de-germinating and other steps involved in most of today's 'enriched'
> bread production results in even greater food value losses, even
> greater incorporation of chemical additives. (The agene process of
> whitening bread with the bleaching agent nitrogen trichloride has been
> established as responsible for producing epilepsy in dogs, identical
> to the human disease.) Most commercial whole wheat breads contain
> even greater amounts of 'freshness extenders', so avoidance of white
> bread alone is not the solution."

Chemical Poisoning of Grain Crops on the Farm

The chemical poisoning of bread starts on the farm. If the grain from
which bread is made was grown on land contaminated by poisonous insecticide
residues, resulting from the spraying of previous crops (and what American
farmlands today have not been so contaminated?), these chemicals will be taken
up by growing plants and will find their way to the wheat or rye that is
harvested from the crop, even if grown in a natural manner without chemicals.
However, this is generally not the case, for chemical fertilizers are used
in the production of all commercial grain crops, and some are sprayed with
DDT or other insecticides.

Another source of chemical contamination of grain are the chemical seed
preservatives with which the seed is treated before planting, in order to
free them from disease-carrying smut and rust organisms. There is reason to
believe that the poison thus applied to seeds definitely penetrates into them
and that some of it will show up in the seed of the new crop used to make
bread. Practically all wheat seed has been treated with a mercury-containing
poison named Ceresan. Wheat seed treated with it is so poisonous that bags in
which it is packed are marked 'caution,' with instructions not to feed it to
farm animals.

There are two ways in which poisonous chemical seed preservatives find
their way into the growing crop. First by direct absorption through the
outer wall of the seed and secondly by being dissolved by soil moisture and
permeating the surrounding soil on which the seedling feeds. The modern
practice of coating seeds with plant nutrients in order to secure better
germination and growth, is an application of the same principle. The only

difference is that in the first case a poison surrounds the seed and is taken up by the seedling and in the latter case plant food is similarly applied and absorbed. In this way, poisonous seed preservatives become part of the future plant's structure and are transmitted to the grain that is formed.

Chemical fertilizers constitute an unquestionable source of soil and food poisoning; and grain crops grown by use of such fertilizers take them up and transmit them to the resulting harvest, whose flavor, quality and nutritive value are thereby lowered. Anyone who has tasted and eaten organically grown grains will distinctly notice their superiority over those grown with chemicals, both in flavor and in health value. Chemical fertilizer residues are unquestionably taken up by plants and transmitted to the grain they produce. Another evil is the use of weed-killing sprays on grain crops; these find their way into the soil, are taken up by the plants, and reappear in the grain they produce.

Fumigation of Grain After Harvesting

But this is only the beginning. After harvesting, grain is fumigated with cyanogen to kill grain weevils and to guard against insect infestation during storage. This poison is so dangerous that the farmer, when applying it, wears a gas mask to protect himself. There is evidence that some quantities of fumigants are absorbed by the grain and communicated to the consumer, exercising a harmful effect. Today practically all grain products, legumes, nuts and seeds sold to the American public have been fumigated, and contain toxic residues derived therefrom. If hard grains, legumes, seeds and nuts absorb and communicate to consumers toxic residues from fumigants, how much more should softer and more absorptive dates, bananas and oranges do so? In the case of dates grown in California, it is a universal practice to fumigate with methyl bromide. Bromides, as is well known, are brain sedatives and constituents of sleeping powders, which have in many cases caused death. Bananas it may be noted in passing, are not only fumigated, but, since the bananas imported to this country are subject to a banana disease, they are sprayed with copper and sulphate, sometimes visible on them as a green powder. This chemical accumulates in the soil in which bananas grow, until it becomes so poisoned that it fails to produce a normal crop. Needless to say, the banana plant absorbs this poison from the soil, and transmits it to the interior of bananas. This must cause the bananas to become diseased and require more spraying. Thus a vicious circle is formed, and the soil becomes more and more poisoned, until it is incapable of producing a crop.

Machine Milling and Refining of Grain

After being subjected to these various forms of chemical contamination on the farm, the next mistreatment that grain receives occurs in the mill. In place of the old-fashioned method of slow stone-grinding by water power, steel rollers are used. These steel rollers cause a destruction of vitamins (through the generation of heat during the milling process), as well as a certain amount of metallic contamination by the wearing away of the machinery. On this subject, P.M. Kourenoff writes:

"Coarse stone-ground flour is more healthful than mill ground flour. Those who eat it rarely have stomach ailments. It is entirely possible that flour ground between steel rollers absorbs microscopic bits of metal due to gradual wearing of the steel under great pressure."

Grain is further contaminated by being refined, its vital germ, which contains most of its vitamins and minerals, being removed and leaving the rest of the grain which consists largely of starch. It has been estimated that while the old fashioned stone-grinding process retained about 75% of vitamin B-1, the white flour of today, which has been machine milled and refined, has only about 10% of this vitamin retained. It is claimed that since the beginning of modern steel-milling and refining of grains, polio and other nervous diseases, digestive disorders, decayed teeth and constipation have been on the steady increase. During the process of refining, the wheat berry is deprived of most of its iron and phosphorus. By removal of its germ it is also deprived of vitamin B Complex and vitamin E. Since the germ is the vital part of the grain and since it quickly deteriorates, by its removal a more stable product is created which may more readily be stored and kept on grocery shelves.

Enrichment with Synthetic Vitamins

After grains have been deprived of their vitamins and minerals by the refining process, synthetic vitamins (coal-tar products) and inorganic iron salts are added in order to enrich it. There are two objections to this practice. The first is that synthetic vitamins manufactured in the chemical laboratory or factory, as shown in the next chapter, cannot replace the natural vitamins removed from grain when refined, either in quality or variety, nor can inorganic iron salts added to flour replace the organic iron present in the whole grain prior to refining. The second objection is that the addition of just a few artificial vitamins and minerals cannot take the place of the much greater variety of vitamins and minerals removed from refined grains. For this reason in some countries, like Canada, the 'enrichment' of bread with synthetic substitutes for the natural vitamins and minerals taken away from it is prohibited by law, which would mean that the practice is considered harmful to the health of consumers. However, in this country, twenty-eight states have laws that make it compulsory for bread to be thus enriched.

Over twenty vitamin and mineral elements are removed from whole wheat when converted into white flour, yet only four or five are thus replaced, and in an inferior, synthetic form, which may do more harm than good. There is considerable evidence that vitamins and minerals in natural organic form, as provided by natural unrefined foods are better that synthetic concentrates, and that organically grown foods are richer in vitamins and minerals than are those grown with or treated with chemicals.

Many experiments have demonstrated the superiority of natural over synthetic vitamins. Referring to the fact that mice with scurvy, when given synthetic forms of vitamin C did not recover, while when given this vitamin in a natural, organic form, they did; Rodale remarks, "It would seem therefore that when synthetic vitamins are thrown into that flour mix, there is a question in my mind how good it is. Inorganic iron salts added to bread are certainly not as good as natural, organic iron compounds removed from grain when refined. (An excess of vitamin B-1, produced synthetically, can produce sterility. The vitamin enrichment of bread can therefore do more harm than good.)"

Bleaching Chemicals - Producers of Insanity

The next source of poisoning the wheat from which our bread is made is the bleaching process, which has been most severely condemned by authorities. In the bleaching of flour, aluminum compounds, ammonia and gypsum (Plaster of Paris), as well as other chemicals, are used, most of which are known to be toxic to human beings.

One of the most common bleaches is nitrogen trichloride or agene. Sir William Mellanby proved that the use of this chemical for bleaching flour caused fits of insanity in dogs, which led to an investigation by the English government on the use of nitrogen trichloride as a bleaching agent, which proved it to be definitely injurious to health.

Regarding the harmful effects of bleaching chemicals, Mellanby wrote: "Some of the increase in the common disorders of the alimentary tract - appendicitis, chloecystitus and peptic ulcer - might possibly be attributed to this large scale tampering with natural foodstuffs." Dr. A.J. Carlson of the University of Chicago called nitrogen trichloride, used for the bleaching of flour, a nerve poison. Dr. William Brady claims that "dogs fed mainly or entirely on white bread or white flour products may develop what is mistaken for rabies - shunning food, losing weight, avoiding light, trembling, cringing when patted, climbing walls, falling backward, howling piteously, falling into their pans if they try to eat and running around madly." In other words, they develop a form of dog insanity.

Psychiatrists claim that bleached flour may contribute to mental diseases. Dr. Schaull of the Stanford University Medical School believes that the tremendous increase of mental diseases among Americans is due in part to eating bread made with bleached flour.

Today, chlorine dioxide is largely used for bleaching flour in this country. This chemical has been found to be definitely toxic to laboratory animals

Chemical Preservatives

Flour is next treated with a disinfecting chemical to kill fungi and bacteria. Mycobahn, or calcium propionate, is used for this purpose. Every atom of the dough mixture is saturated with this chemical. It is known that while calcium propionate resists mold growth, it also destroys the enzyme that enables the body to utilize the small amount of calcium left in white bread; and, like all chemicals added to foods, is harmful.

Since whole wheat, containing the vital germ, is subject to more rapid deterioration than white flour, more chemical preservatives are found in whole wheat bread than in white bread, so that the whole wheat bread sold to the American public is more harmful to health even than white bread. To prevent whole wheat from becoming rancid, about 400 per cent more preservative chemicals are used on it than in the case of white bread. It has been found that such chemically treated whole wheat bread is terribly deadly to experimental animals fed on it.

In evidence of this fact, Wellcome Research Laboratories fed mice with both whole wheat and white bread diets. They were all injected with pneumonia germs. The mice receiving the whole wheat bread died on an average of 1.7 days, while those on the white bread diet survived more than twice as long, namely 3.8 days. Other experiments showed that mice fed whole wheat bread were extinct in 3 generations, while those on white bread were able to wean 54.8 per cent of their young into the third generation. On the basis of such data, J.I. Rodale, editor of "Prevention" and Dr. Royal Lee, of the Lee Foundation for Nutritional Research, both conclude that whole wheat bread, as now available, is definately much more than white bread, as bad as the latter is. This is because it contains more preservative chemicals which are definitely injurious to health.

Chemical Dough Conditioners

The next step in the conditioning of dough by addition of chemical dough conditioners to enable bread to retain its freshness and softness for a longer period without getting stale, while standing on grocer's shelves, as well as to give it a smoother texture and more attractive appearance. The chemical accomplishes this by making the flour absorb more water, in some cases as much as six times its weight. Some of the chemicals used as dough conditioners are similar to the anti-freeze mix used for auto radiators. One of the chemicals used as a dough conditioner is polyexy ethelyne monosterate. Workers in factories where this chemical is made have been known to develop various kinds of skin rashes, even from the fumes. The cumulative effect of daily intake of such chemicals present in baker's bread must be definitely disease-producing in time. Polyexy ethelyne monosterate is also used in the making of peanut butter, ice cream, candy and salad dressings.

Artificial Colorings and Flavorings

Next come the coal tar colorings and flavorings used in bread and cake. Coal tar products are known to be cancer-producing. Some cake decorations contain metallic substances, as aluminum and brass, to give a silver or gold color.

Baking Powder Containing Alum (Aluminum)

Still another harmful chemical added to baked products, crackers, pancake flours, cakes, etc. is baking powder, a strong alkali which destroys the natural hydrochloric acid of the stomach. It is still more dangerous when alum (aluminum) is added to it. For many years a controversy raged between scientists who opposed the addition of aluminum compounds to baking powder, on the ground that it was injurious to the health of consumers, and the aluminum and baking powder companies which favored its use. The opponents of the use of aluminum compounds in baking powder offered some scientific evidence to prove that such aluminum in foods is cancer-producing, as well as causing other serious diseases. However, the vested interests behind the use of aluminum in baking powder were so powerful that they succeeded in silencing the opposing scientists, after a long, drawn out legal suit against the baking powder companies, on the ground that addition of aluminum to baking powder was a menace to public health. (The same occured in the case of Coca Cola, another menace to public health, which, though forbidden to be shipped from state to state, since it violates interstate commerce laws, is permitted to be manufactured and sold within each state.) Baking powders, containing poisonous alum (aluminum) are still permitted to be sold and to render all baked products made with them a potential cause of disease from aluminum poisoning.

Chemical Yeast Food

Yeast, of course, is less dangerous than baking powder, but yeast cells, like other organisms, are as healthy or as unhealthy as is the food on which they feed. It is a common practice to add chemical yeast food to bread, which means the yeast feeds upon chemicals and so cannot be considered as healthful as addition to bread as yeast fed on natural nutrients.

Salt, A Physiological Poison

Still another harmful chemical added to bread is inorganic sodium chloride, commonly known as salt. This is definately a physiological poison, even if it does not kill humans outright, as it does certain lower forms of life, as chickens or pigs, if they swallow enough of it at one time. It differs in no marked manner from other chemical compounds of chlorine, as calcium chloride, magnesium chloride, etc; and while we would regard with abhorrance the addition of these other chemicals, taken from the druggist's shelf, to our foods, we permit and condone the use of salt, merely because the practice is so universal. It is a proven fact that salt injures the kidneys, disturbs the action of the heart muscle, and has a decalcifying effect, due to the property of sodium salts to make calcium more soluble and keep it in solution.

Sugar and refined shortenings and cheap egg and milk substitutes are other sources of the contamination of bread. Even the water with which the dough is mixed may be a source of chemical contamination, due to the presence of chlorine, aluminum, dissolved pipe metals and often poisonous sodium fluoride in city water. Next we must consider possible metallic contamination from the machinery in which the dough is mixed and prepared for the oven - since modern bread is in a real sense a factory product, rather than being hand-made as in former times, when the dough was exposed to much less possibility of metallic contamination by machinery.

We can go on and on and refer to possible contamination when bread is baked in modern gas or electrically heated metallic ovens, rather than in wood-heated brick ovens as was the case years ago, insufficient baking, use of waxed paper wrappers, etc., but enough has been said to prove that bread today is a chemically contaminated product entirely unfit to eat.

How to Make Your Own Alkaline Unleavened Undegerminated Corn and Millet Health Bread

What shall we eat in place of that chemically contaminated product of modern baking industry miscalled 'bread' today - which is definitely a cause of disease? Even at best, wheat is not the best grain. Corn and millet are much better, for while whole wheat is highly acid-forming and decalcifying, these other grains are not. For years the writer has made at home his own unleavened corn and millet bread from organically grown, stone ground cornmeal and millet. These breads were most healthful, delicious and easy to make. Let me explain how.

First obtain a heat-resistant glass distilling apparatus to produce your own supply of glass-distilled water, for it would be ridiculous to make the effort to secure organically grown, stone-ground grains and then contaminate them with chemical and metal containing tap water. Then secure organically grown stone-ground white and yellow cornmeal and millet meal or flour.

To make a delicious, nutritious, digestible, non-fermenting, non-fattening and laxative unleavened whole corn bread, mix one part of yellow cornmeal with two parts of white cornmeal and one part of grated fresh coconut (or coconut meal, if you do not have fresh coconut - or else use sesame seed meal or flaxseed meal, if you wish a more laxative effect.)

Add sufficient glass-distilled water to make a rather watery batter and spread on a glass baking pan which was previously oiled with sesame seed oil, and bake until done. It will be found to be so delicious and so far superior to wheat and rye bread (which are tasteless without the addition of salt and fat, while this corn bread is replete with natural flavor of its own, indicative of its higher mineral content) that you will never care to go back to their use. Also it is much more alkaline on the system than are these acid-forming grains.

To make a super delicious and nutritious organic health cake, follow the same recipe but add organically grown unfiltered maple syrup to sweeten the mixture, also some organically grown chopped dates, seedless raisins, or unfumigated figs, and some ground pistachio or filbert kernels. Sprinkle some pine nut kernals on top. Then put in the oven and bake until done.

A similar bread and cake may be made with millet meal or flour, mixing with white cornmeal if you wish to lighten it, using the latter in place of white flour. Or you may make a millet-corn bread by adding millet meal to the above recipe.

Another way to prepare cornmeal and millet meal is to first cook them as a mush or cereal in a double boiler, together with sesame seed meal, and while hot, pour into an oiled baking dish and place in a cool place until they congeal. Then slice and prepare as patties or bake. The baked sliced cornmeal or millet meal provides an excellent, alkaline, healthful substitute for acid-forming bread of wheat or rye. (While white bread is known to be acid-forming, whole wheat bread was found by tests to be still more acid forming because higher in protein, the source of the uric acid which wheat forms in the body. The same is true of rye which, however, is better than wheat, because richer in minerals and less acid-forming, though inferior to corn and millet.

Pop corn, if organically grown, and popped without salt (using powdered kelp or dulse to satisfy the craving for salt), with virgin sesame seed oil in place of the cheap, more acid-forming oils generally used for making pop corn, is an excellent substitute for bread. Pop corn is laxative since it supplies non-irritating hydroscopic roughage which promotes peristalsis, non fattening (it being starch-free, since during the process of popping, its starch is converted into dextrine, a pre-digested carbohydrate), non-acid-forming and rich in vitamins and minerals. Properly prepared it is a very digestible food, to be recommended to those who suffer from gas after eating fermented bread. Due to its property to absorb moisture, containing acids, in the stomach and intestines, it is an excellent food, in place of acid-forming wheat and rye, for sufferings from acid indigestion, and especially for those allergic to wheat or on reducing diets for obesity.

Organically grown Irish potatoes also provide an excellent, healthful substitute for bread. The superior nutritional virtues of potatoes, if grown without chemicals or sprays, will be described in more detail in a later chapter.

In general, a dish of cornmeal mush or millet, cooked as a cereal, or wild rice (or else brown rice, though wild rice is far superior and worth its extra cost because of its much higher vitamin and mineral content), provide excellent substitutes for bread. Many tropical and oriental races never eat bread, eating a bowl of rice or millet instead. The bread-eating habit is an artificial one, and is often a form of vicarious alcoholism, since fermented bread, in the presence of the hydrochloric acid of the stomach, undergoes a form of alcoholic fermentation, leading to the production of acids and gases, which is most marked in the case of wheat, to which many are allergic for this reason, and should use corn, millet or wild rice instead. (Corn germ, present in all undegerminated cornmeal and popcorn, is far superior to wheat germ as a source of vitamin B complex, essential amino acids and other nutrients including lecithin and vitamin E.

CHAPTER FIVE

NATURAL VERSUS SYNTHETIC VITAMINS

Why Natural Vitamins Are Better Than Synthetic

Every day, more and more people are becoming disillusioned with synthetic vitamins, and are finding that they fail to produce the results claimed for them by the advertising literature of their manufacturers. There is a growing conviction among many scientists that the effects of such vitamins are more psychological than physiological. This conclusion is based on certain experiments performed on groups of individuals who were given pills containing vitamins, while controls were given placeboes, or identical pills without vitamins, both groups being told that they were taking vitamin pills. Observations of the results of such experiments showed that the effects of both kinds of pills, with and without vitamins, were identical. Physiologically, the effects were nil. The experiments indicated that whatever benefits vitamins were supposed to bring about are purely psychological and due to autosuggestion.

The trend today is definitely away from synthetics and in the direction of natural vitamins as present in Organic foods. The public is gradually wakening up to the fact that no chemist in his laboratory can create life, and that since vitamins are so closely associated with life, neither can he create a vitamin as exists in nature. There is increasing scientific evidence accumulating that not only are synthetic vitamins, produced in the chemical laboratory, unable to replace natural vitamins in natural value, but they may actually be harmful. Since they are produced by the action of chemicals (chiefly coal tar and petroleum derivatives) and by treatment with heat, their associated enzymes, which are present in association with natural vitamins, and without which vitamins cannot produce their full physiological effects, have been destroyed. At best they are poor imitations of natural vitamins, even if they have an identical chemical formula. There is more to life than mere chemistry. A living man and a dead man may have the same chemical structure, and so a natural vitamin, as created by nature may have the same formula as an artificial one created by a chemist - yet be entirely different in its effect on the user. The first contains a mysterious quality the latter lacks - which we call 'life'.

Artificial vitamins are of two types - crystalline vitamins, which are derived from natural materials that have been subjected to a chemical and heating treatment, as a result of which they have been reduced to a crystalline form, and synthetic vitamins, which are made from cheap material, such as coal tar derivatives, and which have been synthesized by chemical treatment according to the chemical formula of crystalline vitamins, of which they represent artificial imitations. Neither the crystalline nor the synthetic vitamins contain associated enzymes, as present in natural vitamins, nor the various trace minerals found together with vitamins in living plants, especially sea plants, which are the richest source of trace minerals in the entire vegetable kingdom. Since these enzymes and trace minerals are essential for vitamin metabolism and optimal utilization, it is clear that crystalline and synthetic vitamins cannot replace natural ones.

Why are millions of dollars worth of synthetic vitamins bought each year by the American people - if vitamins do not really produce the results claimed for them? Why, in spite of all the vitamins that the American people buy and use, are they becoming sicker than ever, and why are the more serious chronic degenerative diseases, as heart disease and cancer, on the steady increase? Why are races which live close to nature, subsisting on organically grown foods - as the Hunzas - and who never used a single vitamin or knew that they existed (or the Japanese, who use sea vegetation as a source of vitamins) free from diseases that afflict the vitamin-using Americans? Could it be that the chief cause of vitamin deficiency in this country is the fact that foods are raised on depleted soils, failing to furnish the trace minerals they should, without which plants cannot elaborate vitamins, with the result that animals and humans subsisting on such vitamin-deficient plants suffer nutritional deficiencies as a result?

There are many people today who enjoy excellent health, though they use no vitamin products whatever, obtaining their vitamins entirely from organically grown foods. There can be no doubt that this is the natural and best way to secure vitamins, for Organic Foods provide a nutritional balance of vitamins, enzymes and minerals, in proper proportion and combination. On the other hand, when using artificial vitamins there is a danger of overdosage of certain factors, leading to compensatory deficiency of others, and resulting in nutritional imbalance. For example, studies have shown that an excess of certain vitamin B factors, as thiamin, will lead to a compensatory deficiency of other factors, as pyridoxine. Also, unless vitamins are balanced by a sufficient variety of trace minerals in organic combination, they cannot produce their full effect. Thus, cobalt was found necessary for the proper action of vitamin B-12. But if inorganic cobalt is added to this vitamin, it will not have the same effect as organic cobalt, as provided by sea vegetation. The animal and human organisms were intended by nature to obtain their minerals in organic form, as provided by plants, and cannot directly assimilate or use inorganic minerals, as plants can. Plants are the intermediaries between the inorganic world and the animal world, for which reason we should secure our vitamins and minerals from plants, and not in the form of synthetic creations of the chemical laboratory.

Organic Foods provide a natural complex of vitamins, enzymes, minerals, phosphatides, proteins, carbohydrates and fats in a proper nutritional balance; and hence are far superior as a source of vitamins than synthetic products. More and more progressive people are giving up the use of vitamin products and are using Organic Foods instead.

How Crystalline and Synthetic Vitamins Are Made

How are crystalline vitamins made? They are made of certain natural materials which have been treated with one or more of the following chemical solvents:

   Ether - made from alcohol and sulphuric acid
   Benzine - a petroleum derivative
   Toluene - a coal tar derivative
   Trichlorethyline - a petroleum derivative treated with chlorine gas (a poisonous gas)
   Methylalcohol - a wood alcohol synthetically made

The resultant product is then treated with some precipitant, such as iron chloride, barium chloride, lead salts, aluminum salts, etc. It is then filtered, distilled by heat and then recovered in crystalline form.

Can such a product conceivably bring health to the user? Can such artificial vitamins equal in value the natural vitamins, combined with trace minerals, of Organic Foods? Certainly not! And can isolated synthetic vitamins, created in the chemical laboratory, replace the natural vitamin complex found in Organic Foods in association with closely-bound enzymes, coenzymes, minerals (including trace minerals), proteins, fats and carbohydrates? No! They positively cannot!

Synthetic vitamins are a chemical reconstruction of crystalline vitamins, produced in the manner above described. While the crystalline vitamins are originally derived from natural sources, the synthetic product is made from cheap materials, which are reduced to a chemical formula that is the same as that of the crystalline vitamin. As in the case of the crystalline vitamin, the synthetic vitamin is devoid of associated enzymes, trace minerals, etc., present together with the vitamins of Organic Foods and which are necessary for proper vitamin utilization. Evidently any product artificially created by synthetic chemical combination, in imitation of vitamins as existing in natural foods, by its very nature, cannot provide the enzymes that act with the vitamins, nor furnish the synergizing values of natural vitamins and other factors of Organic Foods.

Synthetic vitamins are often a will o' the wisp, which lead one nowhere. We must get to the cause of vitamin deficiency, and using synthetic vitamins does not remove this cause. The cause is soil depletion of essential of essential minerals needed for the elaboration of vitamins by plants. We must replace these minerals to the soil, grow foods rich in natural vitamins and then consume such mineral and vitamin rich foods. That is the only genuine way to correct nutritional deficiencies - and not the swallowing of pills or capsules purchased over the drug counter. The true solution of the vitamin problem is to comsume a vitamin rich diet of organically grown foods raised on mineral rich soil whose organic life has not been destroyed by the use of chemical fertilizers, which produce bumper crops of poor nutritional value, lacking the vitamins and minerals they should have.

Vitamin Toxicity

There is considerable scientific evidence that synthetic and high potency vitamin concentrates can be toxic. This is because: (1) High doses can act as toxic overdoses, (2) Prolonged intake of coal tar products, from which most synthetic vitamins are made, can be cumulatively toxic, though producing no immediate effects, (3) They can produce allergies, (4) They can be outright toxic, especially when the organism does not need them, as in the case of an absence of deficiencies.

Outright vitamin deficiencies, in this country, are rare. Most common are the borderline, subclinical cases. In such cases overdosage of vitamins may be harmful. An example of toxicity produced by vitamins is afforded by irradiated ergosterol. An overdose can lead to kidney stones, polyurea and other symptoms. It is difficult to determine where overdosage begins.

Too much vitamin A, even when derived from natural sources, can produce toxic symptoms, as weakness, weight loss, nausea, diarrhea, stomach cramps, headaches, stupor, forms of anemia, loss of minerals in bones and blood changes. Chaplin, Clark and Ropes, writing in the <u>American Journal of Medical Sciences</u>, report eleven such cases. A woman poisoned by too much vitamin A was described in the <u>Journal of the American Medical Association</u> by Sulsberger and Lazar. Hearing that vitamin A may prevent catching cold, she began to take 600,000 units per day and kept it up for 18 months. The average person needs only 5,000 units per day, so she was swallowing 120 times her daily requirement, not to mention the vitamins she was getting in foods. She finally came to the doctors because her hair was falling out and her eyebrows and eyelashes were almost gone. She had aches in bones and joints, soreness and cracks in the corners of her mouth, a dry, rough, very itchy skin, with some discolored patches, night sweats and other complaints. In children, too much vitamin A is blamed for causing loss of appetite and weight, irritability, low grade fever, skin rash, loss of hair, enlargement of liver, blood changes and tenderness over the long bones of the body. Gritbetz, Silverman and Sobel, writing in the <u>Pediatrics Journal</u>, report that fourteen similar cases of vitamin A poisoning in infants and children and warn that excess vitamin intake may be as dangerous as deficient intake. Just where the dividing line between normal and excessive intake exists is often difficult to say. For this reason it is safer to secure vitamins in the form of natural foods than in the form of artificial concentrates. An example is afforded by wheat germ oil as a source of vitamin E. This is admitted toxic except in small carefully regulated doses. On the other hand, sesame and sunflower seeds provide an abundance of vitamin E in a safe, natural form, balanced by other factors which minimize danger of overdosage if these seeds are eaten freely.

Most synthetic vitamins are made out of coal tar. It is known that coal tar, even when used externally, can cause cancer of the skin; and when taken internally, it is known to cause internal cancer. In view of these facts, we cannot imagine how synthetic vitamins, made from coal tar, can be anything but harmful to health, even though they may produce no immediate injurious effects that are noticeable. However, Reingold and Webb, in the <u>Journal of the American Medical Association</u>, 1946, 130, 491, reported a case of death resulting from large doses of thiamine, or vitamin B-1, a coal tar product. Riboflavin is another coal tar product: as also is niacin, which can produce variable reactions, such as increases in temperature over the face, ears and neck, with flushing, burning and itching of the skin. Pyridoxine is also a coal tar derivative. Animal experiments have shown that the vitamin possesses high toxicity causing ataxia and convulsions in dosage of one gram. Vitamin G is also synthetically made from coal tar derivatives and in large doses is known to cause anorexia and diarrhea: and in susceptible individuals the reaction is even worse, according to the <u>Journal of Nutrition</u> (August - 1951).

Like synthetic vitamins, synthetic inorganic minerals, often added to vitamins, are known to be toxic. For example, ferrous sulfate, one of the most popular iron salts used, can cause severe digestive upsets, even in small doses, in many cases. The <u>Journal of the American Medical Assoc.</u> reported a case of death in a child which took a bottle of ferrous sulfate iron tablets, which it mistook for candy. It is known that the body cannot assimilate inorganic minerals, chemicals or drugs, but only minerals in organic form, as provided by plants; and inorganic minerals, for this reason, are harmful. Inorganic iron salts, it is known, cannot be used for hemoglobin formation, as organic iron compounds can be.

A Farm That "Grows" Natural Vitamins on Seaweed-Mineralized Soil

The Hillcrest Nutritional Farm near Kansas City, which is the largest organic farm in the country, covering 472 acres, is devoted to the production of natural vitamins secured from plants grown on special mineral-enriched soil. Here a team of soil scientists and nutritionists have established a unique experiment and a new method of vitamin manufacture. The method consists in growing young tender cereal grasses on soil enriched with organic matter and a vast variety of trace minerals obtained from seaweed. Scientists tested and re-tested the soil of this farm in an attempt to bring it to the optimal level of productivity, not only of crops in large quantity, but also of the highest possible <u>quality</u> - a matter that agriculturists of the past have neglected to consider.

Experiments were conducted, using organic composts with and without seaweed. In every case it was found that seaweed, which provides up to 92 different minerals present in ocean water, (only a part of which have yet been identified by the analytical chemist, who lacks methods fine enough to detect many of the trace minerals that exist therein only in very minute amounts) proved to be the magic spark that provided life-giving nutrients to the soil and to the plants that grew thereon.

This mysterious property of seaweed as a soil conditioner and plant food becomes readily understandable when we consider that for centuries the waters of the earth have washed into the sea minerals leached from the soil, which makes the ocean a veritable treasure chest of minerals washed off the land. As the land-areas of the earth's surface grew poorer and poorer and poorer in minerals, the sea became richer and richer, and so did the plants growing therein. Seaweed, therefore, contains trace minerals that have long since disappeared from land areas, yet which are essential to life. The result is that land-grown plants fail to contain them because the soil on which they grow no longer has them, but in sea plants they are present in comparative abundance. Trace minerals are of utmost importance both to plants and human beings; and most foods in common use lack them. Experiments at the Hillcrest Nutritional Farms have shown that trace minerals are necessary for the production of maximum quantities of vitamins in foods and that seaweeds are the best organic sources of trace minerals. That is why this farm is today the country's largest agricultural user of seaweed as a fertilizer. It is shipped in by the carload from Maine, to give the "magic spark" to the composts used to fertilize the soil. This humus-and-trace-mineral-enriched soil has been found to produce plants of exceptionally high mineral and vitamin content: ORGANIC SUPER FOODS. The important and essential trace minerals that most soils have lost centuries ago and which have been drained into the sea, have, on this farm, been restored to the soil and to foods. Since these trace minerals are the mother-sources of vitamins, we can understand why the Organic Super Foods raised on this farm are so unusually high in vitamins. This farm stands as a shining light and a pioneer of the new Organic Age in nutrition, when natural vitamins, produced on the soil, in the fresh air and sunshine, will replace the synthetic products of the chemical laboratory.

On this wonderfully enriched soil, oats, wheat, barley, rye and corn were planted. These grains were not left to mature, but when the young, tender cereal sprouts were a few days old, they were harvested. It was determined that at this time they were at the height of their vitality content. The fresh, natural juices of these cereal sprouts were then concentrated, and, by a special method, and reduced to a powdered form. While old-fashioned methods of dehydration involved a high temperature that killed vitamins and minerals, the dehydration of these young cereal grasses took place at a rather low temperature, so as to preserve the precious enzymes and vitamins. The result was a powdered concentrate of the juice of young cereal grasses, which contained, in natural form and combination, vitamins in combination with minerals, enzymes and other elusive food factors. This product heralds a new era in nutrition - NATURAL VITAMINS DERIVED FROM ORGANIC FOODS GROWN ON SOIL ENRICHED BY SEAWEED-MINERALIZED COMPOSTS. Such vitamin products created by Nature are destined to replace the old synthetic and crystalline vitamins.

CHAPTER SIX

TRACE MINERALS AND SEA VEGETATION

In the last chapter we have seen that the plants of the sea are the richest sources of trace minerals in the plant world. We have also pointed out that these trace minerals play an essential role in both plant and animal metabolism, and that unless they are supplied to the soil in sufficient amounts, plants will be unable to elaborate optimal quantities of vitamins. Nor can they supply us with these trace minerals, which are so essential to our health and well being. Indeed, these much-neglected trace minerals, about which we know so little, yet which are so important, seem to hold the secret of successful nutrition. Most soils lack them; most foods contain little or none of them; and most people suffer a deficiency of them, usually without knowing it. Yet Nature has provided us with a plentiful supply of trace minerals in the plants of the sea. Sea plants are undoubtedly the richest and best possible sources of all essential vitamins and minerals in natural organic form. This is proven by the excellent physiques of Polynesian and Oriental races which incorporate a variety of edible seaweed in their diet, and who are free from vitamin deficiencies though they never take any vitamins - indeed, freer than we are, in spite of all the artificial vitamins we consume! For it is a fact that it is from the minerals of the soil - especially the trace minerals - that plants elaborate vitamins. And since sea plants obtain from trace minerals their nutrient medium, we can understand why they are far richer in vitamins than land-grown vegetation.

Concerning the physiological significance of trace minerals, *Normal Agriculture* (January 1953) writes: "The surface has been scratched on a few of these trace elements - manganese, cobalt, copper, iron, molybdenum, zinc and boron. But there are sixty-some others - everything from antimony to zirconium. Where do they fit into the nutritional picture?"

"One hint of the many indications of the importance of trace elements had come from the findings of an independent Danish investigator, Ottar Rygh...Rygh had discovered five elements that are concerned with the body's use of calcium: strontium, vanadium, zinc, barium and thallium, the first two tending to promote calcification, with the latter three aiding decalcification. The trace element field in nutrition studies is wide open."

Let us consider some of the important trace minerals required by the body, which are abundant in sea vegetation, but which tend to be lacking in most land-grown foods:

COBALT. This mineral, present in sea vegetation, is closely related to the anti-anemic vitamin B-12. It has been found to act in conjunction with iron, copper and manganese in hemoglobin formation and regeneration. Some persistent human nutritional anemias refuse to clear up completely when iron alone is given, but disappear when cobalt is added. There is a lack of cobalt in most land-grown foods.

COPPER. This mineral is also present in sea vegetation, but tends to be lacking in most land-grown foods. Since the animal body cannot form red blood cells and hemoglobin in the absence of copper, or forms them at a very slow rate, it is clear that copper is as important as iron for hemoglobin formation. It is believed that copper and cobalt aid the assimilation of iron and work with iron in overcoming anemia.

FLUORINE. This trace mineral, essential for the building of tooth enamel, is present in sea vegetation, which provides it in a safe organic form, much better than in the inorganic form, as provided by sodium fluoride, a rat poison added to drinking water, under the mistaken idea that this is equivalent to organic fluorine, which it is not. For the body can assimilate minerals only in organic combination, and not in inorganic form. When inorganic fluorides are taken in drinking water, rather than entering into the composition of normal tooth enamel, they tend to cause mottling of the teeth, having a harmful effect, as all inorganic chemicals do. Much better it would be to add some sea vegetation to one's diet if one desires extra fluorine, and not to practice mass medication by adding poisonous inorganic sodium fluoride to city water supplies.

BROMINE. This is an interesting trace mineral present in the ocean, in sea vegetation and in sea air. It is closely related to iodine, and, like iodine, is important for the brain. As important as iodine is for the thyroid gland, bromine is important for the pituitary gland. The pituitary gland contains 7 to 10 times as much bromine as any other organ of the body. It is known that in certain forms of insanity, known as manic-depressive psychoses, the normal blood bromine is reduced to about one half. During old age, the amount of bromine in the brain diminishes. After 45 it starts to fall and at 75 there is only a trace of bromine, if any, in the brain. Coincident with this loss of bromine by the brain, there is a diminution of brain energy and efficiency. In senile dementia, the bromine content of the brain is very low. All this indicates the value of the addition of sea vegetation to the diet to supply sufficient bromine, as well as iodine, both of which minerals are important for the normal well-being of the brain and the prevention of brain decline in old age. Sufficient is also important for optimal nutrition of the pituitary gland. Bromine tends to be deficient in land-grown plants, but is abundant in sea vegetation.

IODINE. Without iodine, the brain cannot work, nor can it develop normally. Iodine is needed by the thyroid gland for the manufacture of its hormone thyroxin, which contains brain activity. Thyroxin appears to act as a catalyst that activates the oxidation of phosphorus compounds (lecithin) in the brain cells, which generates currents of brain electricity on which the functioning of these cells, manifesting in human intelligence, depends. For this reason, children born with congenitally defective thyroid glands never develop normally in their mental growth, as is the case in cretinism, a form of idiocy due to thyroid undevelopment and incapacity to supply the brain with its iodine-containing hormone.

It is well known that the soils of certain regions are so deficient in minerals that animals feeding thereon cannot grow and reproduce normally. One of these is iodine, which is lacking in soils remote from the sea, which is the source of this element, which is distributed over land areas by wind-borne sea spray. This results in iodine deficiency diseases in such regions, such as the hairless pig malady among animals (incapacity of pigs to reproduce normal offspring) and cretinism and goiter among humans, which are common in inland regions as the "goiter" belt of the central states of the United States and in Switzerland. These diseases result from lack of iodine in soil and foods. Administration of sodium iodide or iodized salt to inhabitants of such regions cannot solve the problem, since the body is not able to assimilate iodine in inorganic form, no more than it can assimilate fluorine of any other mineral. Goiter is practically unknown in Japan where sea vegetation, rich in organic iodine, is consumed daily as a part of the diet; and this is the best way to obtain iodine and counteract iodine deficiency diseases. Addition of kelp meal to the feed of animals has proven extremely beneficial, resulting in improved growth and better health, by supplying them with trace minerals most soils and foods grown thereon, lack. The same occurs when seaweed is used as a fertilizer, which has been practiced by many races since time immemorial. Foods so grown possess exceptionally high vitamin and mineral content. We have already mentioned its use at the Hillcrest Nutritional Farm, devoted to the production of natural vitamin concentrates made from the dehydrated juices of young cereal grasses that were grown with seaweed fertilizer. It is a fact that vegetables grown near the seacoast have a much higher iodine content than the same vegetables grown at a distance from the sea, which makes it clear that inland soils and food products grown thereon will be greatly benefitted by addition of marine trace minerals in the form of seaweed used as fertilizer.

The remarkable transformation of a cretinous idiot (cretinism being a disease of iodine deficiency affecting the thyroid gland, which fails in its capacity to produce its brain-activating hormone, thyroxin) into an apparently normal individual, almost miraculously, by administration of iodine-containing thyroid hormone, indicates the profound influence of iodine on the brain and on thinking processes, just as does the reversion of the individual to his former idiotic state soon after administration of iodine in the form of thyroid hormone is discontinued. Iodine seems to act as an organic catalyst, activating brain cell activity.

The thyroid hormone has a detoxifying action, helping to counteract intestinal putrefaction, for which reason a sufficient intake of iodine is necessary to help the body to destroy putrefactive organisms and to insure normal elimination. And inversely, intestinal putrefaction of animal proteins (meat, fish, fowl, eggs, etc.) tends to irritate and strain the thyroid gland and is one cause of hyperthyroidism (goiter). McCarrison, in his studies on goiter, has shown that acid-forming fats drawing iodine from active use by the thyroid gland. It is well known that meat is bad for the thyroid and is counterindicated in thyroid conditions, especially when the thyroid is overactive, as in goiter.

Another physiological function of iodine is its capacity to aid in the more effective digestion, assimilation and combustion of fat. One of the characteristic signs of thyroid deficiency is obesity, or tendency of fat to be improperly oxidized and to accumulate in the body. For this reason persons with overactive thyroids tend to be lean, since the iodine-containing thyroid hormone tends to burn up fat. For this reason use of sea plants has been recommended to obese persons to help them reduce.

77.

It may be noticed that obesity is rare among the Japanese and Polynesians who use seaweed as a steady part of their diet. Addition of seaweed to the diet means a plentiful supply of iodine which enables the body to more effectively oxidize and burn up fats.

Iodine seems also necessary for the health and the skin and hair, preventing a dry, wrinkled and coarse skin, as well as falling hair, which are common symptoms of iodine and thyroid deficiency.

While sea vegetation is the most reliable source of iodine, a few land-grown foods contain small amounts of this mineral, especially those growing near the sea, as does the coconut, which seems to require marine trace minerals for its normal growth and well-being, since the coconut palm will not grow when too far away from the sea, whose minerals are conveyed to it through the air, rainfall and subterranean seepage. For this reason coconuts and coconut milk are good sources of iodine and other trace minerals. The same is true of another tropical plant - the pineapple. Among vegetables, their iodine content depends entirely on where they are grown, whether near or far from the sea. A vegetable that is very rich in iodine when grown near the seacoast will be extremely poor or even lacking in iodine when grown in inland regions. In general, the onion family, including garlic, is richer in iodine than most other vegetables. However, no land-grown plant can compare with sea vegetation in richness in iodine.

MANGANESE. This mineral is important for the pituitary gland, which controls mammary functions. This may explain why, when manganese is lacking in the diet of female animals, they completely lose the maternal instinct, and fail to nurse their young. This probably results from defective pituitary functioning, due to lack of this mineral. It is also claimed that without sufficient manganese in the diet, sterility occurs in the male, since the pituitary hormone controls the activity of the gonads. Manganese has been found in the liver, pancreas and adrenal gland and is believed to be necessary for normal bone development and hemoglobin formation. Peppermint and potatoes rank as high amount land-grown plants in manganese content, though this will depend on the manganese content of the soil, which may be increased by use of trace-mineral-containing powdered rock fertilizers, as granite, colloidal phosphate (derived form decomposed bones of prehistoric marine life), etc. But in general, sea vegetation is the richest source of manganese, as it is of other trade minerals.

SILICON. This trace mineral is lacking in most land-grown foods, but is present in sea vegetation. It is important for the normal formation of the hair and nails. It is also important for the pancreas, with whose functioning it appears to be intimately related. Silicon, and zinc are all found in high concentration in the pancreas.

NICKEL. Its exact physiological function is yet unknown. It is found in greatest quantity in the pancreas. It is present in sea vegetation.

BORON. This trace mineral, found in sea vegetation, is important for plant life, and without it, plants will not grown normally. It is believed to be important for animal life, but its exact function is unknown.

This page was omitted in the original book.

opinion that all minerals that were originally in the earth's crust, including those no longer present, and which have long since been washed into the sea, play an important physiological function, of which, in the case of most of them, science is yet unaware. But just as many minerals, as copper, cobalt, etc., which were formerly not believed to have any biological significance, have later been found to be essential to life, so, he claims, the various trace minerals - in fact all the minerals known to chemistry - may some day be recognized to be important for life, nutrition and health. Since sea vegetation contains most or possibly all of these minerals, known and unknown, whether detected in them or yet undetected, Dr. Page advised the incorporation of sea vegetation in the diet to supply the essential trace minerals, known and unknown.

The Japanese people add a wide variety of edible sea plants to their diet. It claimed by authorities that were it not for their use of sea plants, supplying minerals and vitamins that the products of their exhausted soil fail to supply, the Japanese race would have been extinct long ago.

In this country, largely due to the ruinous effects of chemical fertilizers, soil depletion is common too. In United States Senate Document No. 264, we read: The alarming fact is that foods, fruits and vegetables and grains now being raised on millions of acres of land no longer contain enough of certain needed minerals, and are starving us - no matter how much we eat..No man of today can eat enough fruits and vegetables to supply his system with the mineral salts he requires for perfect health because his stomach isn't big enough to hold them."

Since lack of minerals in the soil prevents plants from elaborating the quantity of vitamins that they should, they fail to supply sufficient vitamins to animals and humans that feed on the products of such mineral-poor soil, with resulting deficiency diseases. Addition of seaweed fertilizer to the soil or sea vegetation to the diet will promptly correct this deficiency by supplying the missing vitamins and minerals.

SEA VEGETATION AS SUPER SOURCES OF TRACE MINERALS AND VITAMINS

A government document says in part..."an oil extracted from certain drifted seaweed contained 1,000 times more vitamins A and D than an equal quantity of cod liver oil. This discovery verifies the opinion of many scientists that the vitamins of fish are originally produced by sea plants and then assimilated with the reception of food and stored mainly in the liver. Though it seems premature at this time to make any suggestion as to the utilization of seaweed for vitamin products, it is important to continue these investigations."

Since the capacity of a plant to manufacture vitamins depends on the amount of minerals it receives, we can well understand why sea vegetation, growing in the richest "soil" in the world - ocean water - which contains about 92 different minerals, including trace minerals that land-grown plants lack, should be so extraordinarily rich in vitamins. We have reason to believe, on the basis of the limited vitamin essays made on sea sea vegetation by the U.S. Department of Fisheries, that sea plants are able to supply large amounts of ALL essential vitamins, both known and unknown, and in a much better form than is provided by synthetic products, for not only are the vitamins of sea plants organic, but they exist in a proper and natural combination with each other and with trace minerals that are so important for vitamin assimilation and utilization. Several outstanding nutritional authorities in their recent writings credit sea vegetation as being one of the richest natural sources all essential vitamins. This appears to be born out by the government publication referred to above, which carries a report of a biological assay made by a scientist associated with a government project.

Since the land surface of the earth, as a result of the leaching effect of rainfall, during the course of centuries, in carrying soil minerals, through rivers and streams, into the sea, tends to become poorer and poorer in minerals, while the ocean tends to become richer and richer, we can understand why sea vegetation is so extremely rich in vitamins, while land grown vegetation tends to be deficient, this deficiency tending on the location, since in different regions, different types of soil mineral deficiency occur, whereas the ocean, on the other hand, has a constant mineral composition in all its parts. It is this extreme variability in soil composition that is fundamentally responsible for the widespread vitamin and mineral deficiencies of humans, which constitute a basic cause of disease.

Since foods grown on mineral deficient soils lack minerals and vitamins, with the result that persons who subsist on such foods suffer deficiency diseases, and since this condition is universal in this country, we can understand why the sale of vitamins has developed into a multi-million dollar business, as people sought to obtain in this way the missing elements which the soil and the foods they consumed failed to supply. However, use of artificial, synthetic vitamins failed to solve the problem, since it did not eliminate the fundamental cause - the fact that foods failed to supply them with the vitamins they should contain because the soil on which they grew lacked a sufficient quantity and variety of minerals (including trace minerals) from which plants form vitamins. The soil lacked these minerals because they were washed into the sea during the course of centuries. Since the plants that grow in the sea contain these missing dietary essentials, it would seem more sensible to add sea plants to one's diet and so enrich land grown foods with elements they lack, than to use artifical vitamins manufactured in the chemical laboratory, because they supply vitamins in organic combination with trace minerals and enzymes, all of which are essential for their best physiological effects. Proof of the superiority of sea vegetation over artificial man-made vitamins is afforded by the splendid health and physiques of the pacific races which use various seaweeds in their diet, yet who use no vitamins, and who are free from many of the deficiency diseases to which vitamin-using Americans are subject.

Are Chemical Fertilizers a Cause of Vitamin and Mineral Deficiency?

One reason for the lack of vitamins and minerals in American foods is the universal practice of using chemical fertilizers in their production. Chemical fertilizers, being more soluble than natural soil mineral colloids, tend to replace them in the plant's metabolism, yet they are not capable of being transformed into vitamins by plants as can the natural colloidal minerals of the soil. The result is that plants grown with chemicals are vitamin deficient: and this makes them unhealthy and subject to disease and insect pests. Keens in England has shown that plant diseases of various kinds, including cancer like diseases, have increased by leaps and bounds since the chemical fertilizers were first introduced in agriculture about a century ago; and the same was true of animals and humans that fed on these vitamin-deficient plants. While chemically fertilized plants undergo a rapid growth and develop large-sized tissues, they fail to take up from the soil the natural mineral colloids they should obtain, and in their place contain chemical fertilizer derivatives, incapable of being transformed into the organic minerals and vitamins necessary for the health of animals and humans that feed on them.

Commenting on the fact that foods grown today with chemicals do not have the nutritional value they had in former times when grown naturally, Dr. Alexis Carrel, in his "Man the Unknown", writes: "The staple foods may not contain the same nutritive substances as in former times. Mass production has modified the composition of wheat, eggs, milk, fruit and butter, although these articles have retained their familiar appearance. Chemical fertilizers, by increasing the abundance of crops without replacing the exausted minerals of the soil, have indirectly contributed to change the nutritive value of cereal grains and vegetables. Hens have been compelled, by artificial diet and mode of living, to enter the ranks of mass producers. Has not the quality of their eggs been modified? The same question may be asked about milk, because cows are now confined to the stable all year round, and are fed on manufactured provender. Hygienists have not paid sufficient attention to the genesis of disease."

Chemical fertilization has combined with soil erosion to progressively demineralize the soil, resulting in the mineral and vitamin deficiencies of modern foods and the widespread diseases and degenerations among plants, animals and humans that result from this deficiency. Once more must land creatures return to the sea for their regeneration. At least 400,000,000 of the world's inhabitants have instinctively realized this fact and have added various edible seaweeds to their diet; and so they were able to survive in a state of good health, whereas otherwise they would have perished. Of the 110 different species of marine flora found growing in the Hawaiin waters, about 70 are used for food by the natives. About 35 varieties are used as part of their diet by the Chinese and Japanese. The Irish and many other races use sea vegetation as part of their diet. Many of these sea plants have mucilaginous properties (as is the case with Irish moss), which have great value in counteracting constipation. Others, like agar agar, supply intestinal bulk by their power to absorb and hold water, and hence aid intestinal elimination. Races that use seaweed as part of their diet, for this reason, are comparatively free from constipation and autointoxication. Another reason for this is that sea vegetation is rich in iodine, which promotes better thyroid functioning; and the thyroid hormone has a detoxifying effect on the gastro-intestinal tract, helping to maintain it in a state of healthful functional activity.

Sea vegetation is generally regarded as a "gland food". That this is true is indicated by their richness in iodine, bromine and other minerals needed by the endocrine glands. When the glands do not obtain sufficient of the trace minerals they require they tend to function abnormally or may degenerate. And since land-grown foods tend to lack one or more of these minerals, the importance of adding sea vegetation to insure an adequate supply of these trace minerals for the endocrine glands is obvious.

From time immemorial, edible sea plants have played an important part in the daily diet of the Chinese and Japanese, who usually consume about five or more different varieties at a single meal. These sea plants are very tasty and nutritious when properly prepared in combination with other foods. They are too rich in minerals and vitamins to eat by themselves. Our organisms, through our racial heredity, have adapted themselves, during the course of countless centuries, to a vitamin - and mineral-poor land-grown diet, and are unaccustomed to the intake of such massive amounts of vitamins and minerals which sea plants supply. For this reason they are not appealing when eaten alone, but should be used as supplements to replace the deficiencies of other foods, adding flavor as well as vitamin and mineral nutrients, and in a much better form than synthetic concentrates manufactured in the chemical laboratory. Oriental races which include sea plants as a regular part of their diet are noted for their unusual physical capacity and endurance; as we have already noted in the case of Polynesian races.

Dr. Josephine Tilden of Minnesota University reports that she had the good fortune of living for a time in Tahiti while the natives where living on a diet consisting largely of fruits, vegetables and sea foods including marine algae and rimu. The people were vigorous in body and mind, handsome and healthy, and had perfect teeth. Another visit to the island was made after pastry shops and ice cream wagons had been introduced into this paradise. The bad effects of the foreign diet was immediately apparent. Tahitian children today have soft, crumbling and badly decayed teeth.

Another race that enjoys exceptional health and freedom from disease, including almost complete immunity from tooth decay, lives on the Islands of Aran off the coast of Scotland. These islands have a solid rock surface devoid of trees, shrubbery and soil. There are three islands, each containing about 500 inhabitants. The scanty diet of these islanders consists chiefly of potatoes grown in spacious beds of seaweed composts packed tightly in sunken rocks that have been hollowed out, the tightly packed seaweed being covered with a top surface of decomposed sea plants, providing a complete fertilizer. These people eat no grains of any kind. They have been cited by McCollum as an example of the decalcifying action of grains and the superiority of potatoes as a carbohydrate, in protecting the teeth from decay.

Sea plants take the place of vegetables in the diet of these people. Potatoes and sea vegetation constitute the basis of their diet. Certain varieties of sea plants are eaten raw in salads and others are cooked in soup or mashed in potatoes. The daily bill of fare of these people always includes a salad composed of edible sea plants. On this meager diet, these people are strong, wiry and healthy, and all have good, strong teeth.

In an interesting book "Farming the Bottom of the Sea for Longer Life Through Better Diet", West points out that plants that grow in the ocean contain a wealth of nutrients, whose resources have as yet scarcely been tapped. They supply vitamins and minerals in a far superior form than do man-made synthetic products of chemistry. He claims that science could with great profit study the nutritive value of the plant life of the ocean as sources of vitamins and minerals not found in plants grown on land, or found in negligible amounts.

The Pernicious Salt-Eating Addiction

The eminent German biochemist Bunge has pointed out that most soils tend to be deficient in sodium, which element is easily washed out by rainfall and carried to the sea, where it accumulates, for which reason the ocean and its products contain an excess of sodium, while the land areas and its plants contain an excess of potassium. On this basis he sought to explain the craving of animals and humans for salt, pointing out also that while potassium predominates in the muscular tissues of the body, sodium is present in higher concentration in the blood, so that animals that feed on a herbivorous diet, and do not consume the blood of other animals, have greatest desire for salt. However, the idea that inorganic sodium chloride can satisfy this craving is false. As for the much exploited idea of animals frequenting salt licks in order to obtain the salt they need, which has been frequently advanced by defenders of the unnatural salt-eating habit, the truth is that when animals do so, they usually suffer from a mineral deficiency caused by feeding on sloping, eroded land, which they vainly try to correct in this manner, just as calcium-starved cows or pregnant women may swallow chalk or wall plaster in an attempt to secure this mineral. Whole races of people have been known who never knew what salt was and who never ate it. The Eskimaux eat no salt. Salt-eating is a habit, not a physiological necessity; and a bad one, which is destructive of health.

In spite of the fact that inorganic sodium chloride (common salt) cannot supply the body with the organic sodium it needs, we must agree with Bunge that land-grown plants tend to lack this mineral in which sea vegetation is rich, and that the craving of animals and humans for this missing element should be satisfied - not by the use of salt, but by addition of sea vegetation to their diet. (We do not recommend sea salt, which is another form of inorganic sodium chloride. Instead we recommend sea greens containing organic sodium chloride, using them after their adhering inorganic salt has been washed off.

There is considerable scientific evidence that the salt-eating habit is harmful to health and a cause of disease, since sodium chloride, like potassium chloride, calcium chloride, and other _chemicals_ (for inorganic sodium chloride, or salt, is a _chemical_, not a food, strange as this idea may seem), cannot be used by the body and acts as a foreign impurity, which, when taken in excess, may become a poison. Prof. Sherman of Columbia University has demonstrated that the body cannot use salt, because soon after a meal containing salt, practically all of it was found given off in the urine, in its original form, showing that the body, unable to use it and in order to promptly get rid of this offending and harmful substance, excreted it. This explains the characteristic thirst which salt-eating calls forth, this being an expression of the body's effort to secure extra fluids in order to wash out and get rid of salt as soon as possible. The same occurs in the case of the edema, or water-logging of tissues, which salt is known to cause, this being a protective measure of the body to surround salt accumulations with sufficient fluid, to dilute the concentration of this toxic substance, so that it may do less injury to surrounding cells.

All salt consumed must pass through the delicate kidney tubules in order to be eliminated, and this causes injury to them. For this reason use of salt is forbidden to sufferers from nephritic contitions; and if salt is harmful to the diseased kidney, it should also be injurious to the healthy one, just as any chemical is, and should, if taken daily over a long period of time, predispose to kidney disease and degeneration. The same is true of the heart, for which reason heart specialists recommend salt-free diets to sufferers from cardiac conditions, who are even forbidden to eat ordinary bread due to the small amount of salt in it, and to use instead salt-free bread. Leo Loeb has shown that the action of the heart muscles is controlled by the balance of sodium and calcium salts in the blood, the former exciting them and the latter depressing or contracting them. This would mean that free use of salt must tend to unbalance the normal rhythm of heart muscle activity, leading to palpitation and high blood pressure, in which condition use of salt is known to be very harmful. In recent years a salt-free diet, consisting of rice and distilled water, has been found very effective in the treatment of heart diseases. As in the case of the kidney, if salt is bad for the diseased heart, it should also be bad for the healthy one, and tend to make it diseased.

Persons who are victims of the salt-eating addiction, in order to break themselves from this evil, health-destroying habit, will do well to commence by sprinkling powdered kelp on their foods. This has a salty taste due to its content of sea salt, and will satisfy the desire for salt in a much better way than ordinary salt, without being so harmful, since it supplies both inorganic sodium chloride of sea salt and the organic sodium chloride of the kelp leaf. It will be then good to advance to the use of powdered dulse, which has less sea salt and more organic sodium chloride, and later use the whole dulse leaf, after washing to remove adhering sea salt, so that the body may satisfy its craving for sodium with the _organic_ sodium chloride of the dulse leaf alone. After this one can use various washed Japanese sea greens cooked with one's food. These impart a delicious flavor, and also considerable organic sodium chloride to gratify the craving for this element, which will at the same time reduce the desire for salt. In this way, it will be possible to completely break oneself of the pernicious salt-eating habit, and replace intake of _inorganic_ sodium chloride, in the form of common salt, by _organic_ sodium chloride, in the form of washed sea greens. (The Japanese are so careful to remove all inorganic sea salt from their sea vegetation before using that they carefully rinse it in as many as a dozen changes of water, in order to remove all the sea salt possible.) It is a fact that sodium tends to interfere with the utilization of calcium by keeping this mineral in solution, and is therefore strongly decalcifying. For this reason, it is important to carefully remove all excess salt from sea vegetation before using and prefer the salt-free types (as washed Japanese sea greens) to the salt-containing ones, as powdered kelp and dulse), for otherwise one might obtain a wealth of nearly all other minerals, including an excess of sodium, while at the same time suffering from a compensatory calcium deficiency.

Varieties of Sea Vegetation for Culinary Purposes

Orientals and Pacific islanders are not the only races which add sea vegetation to their diet. The Irish also do, since Irish moss and dulse, commonly known as Irish sea lettuce, grow plentifully along the coast of

Ireland and are used by its inhabitants. Irish moss is valuable for its mucilaginous properties, for which it has long been used as a laxative; and, in powdered form, it is used for making jellies. Irish sea lettuce is a tender greens which may be used raw in salads, giving them a tang and zest that no other additive can equal, besides enriching them with iodine and other valuable trace minerals that land-grown foods lack. One writer on nutrition has accounted for the superior and quicker mentalities of the Irish as due to their use of sea plants supplying them with plenty of iodine for the production of optimal quantities of brain-activating thyroid hormone, whereas the English, who eat no sea vegetation, do not obtain so much iodine in their diet.

Leaf dulse has the advantage over Japanese sea greens in being so tender (tenderer than the tenderest lettuce, after the sea greens are washed to remove adhering sea salt), that it can be eaten raw with other foods (salads, cereals, vegetables, added to soups, etc.) or cooked with them, to enrich them with organic sodium chloride, to place salt. Those who give up the use of salt and find foods tasteless without it will do well to use dulse, both raw and cooked with foods, to season them in its place. After one adds sea plants to one's diet and observes the beneficial effects of their content of trace minerals which most foods lack, one finds them so essential that when their use is suddenly discontinued, foods seem flat and valueless without them. In fact, one becomes as addicted to their use, as the salt-eater is to salt, though in this case it is a healthful and beneficial addiction, resulting from the awakening of a hidden hunger for trace minerals for which one may have been starving all one's life without knowing it, until one commenced to add sea vegetation to one's diet and become conscious of this deficiency.

As we have indicated, to overcome the salt-eating habit, one should commence with powdered kelp and dulse and advance to leaf dulse and Japanese sea greens. The latter are used cooked with other foods, to enrich them with flavor, vitamins and minerals. An excellent one to start with is known as "Oboro Kombu", which is soft white sea plant which comes neatly packaged in cardboard boxes. Within a few minutes after addition to cooked foods while cooking, it swells greatly and becomes mucilaginous. It imparts a delicious flavor and somewhat salt-like taste to food. "Tororo Kombu" is a similar variety, only semi-powdery in consistency, and may be added raw to various foods. It is much better than powdered kelp in being without any strong salty taste, as kelp has, and better for those who wish to avoid salt. (The word "kombu" means kelp in Japanese, most of the Japanese sea greens being varieties of kelp that grow off the coast of Japan.) Another edible sea plant which is a favorite among the Japanese, and which is also available in this country, is "Dashi Kombu". This is a thick-leafed variety of kelp which is used cooked with other foods. As in the case of most dried Japanese sea greens it is prepared by first breaking the leaf into small pieces, then rinsing repeatedly to remove sea salt and then soaking until the pieces of leaf swell to maximum volume. This plant gives off a valuable, beneficial mucilaginous substance into the water, which should be carefully kept and added to foods with which it is cooked, since it has a soothing action on the gastro-intestinal lining, valuable for conditions of inflammation and acting as an intestinal lubricant. As in the case of other

Japanese sea greens used cooked, it is best to use it in limited quantities, combined with much larger amounts of land-grown foods. The reason for this is that sea vegetation is so extremely rich in vitamins and minerals that we, being land creatures, by heredity are not accustomed to such a plentiful intake, which may be overwhelming, so that sea plants, like vitamin and mineral concentrates, as best used as supplements to other foods, rather than as foods in themselves.

"Nishime Kombu" is the name of another Japanese sea plant which resembles "Dashi Kombu", except that the leaf is smaller and thinner and easier to cook. (The cooking time of most Japanese sea plants is less than that of ordinary foods, though their is no harm to cook them with the latter for the same period of time.) "Shiroita Kombu" is another still thinner and more quick-cooking variety of kelp used added to other foods. It is quite gelatinous. "Hijiki" is a Japanese sea plant in the form of small black shreds which enlarge and elongate when soaked, then becoming tender enough to add raw to salads, or they may be added to soup like noodles. "Wakame" is another sea green that somewhat resembles a garden greens when cooked. "Asakusa Nori" is a sea plant delicacy in Japan, which is lowest in salt and ideal for those on salt-free diet. It is eaten by first holding over a flame for a few seconds until it toasts crisp, and then eating. It is very rich in minerlas. Those suffering calcium deficiency would do well to prefer it, due to its low sodium content. On the other hand, sufferers from arthritis and calcareous deposits will do well to use the others that are higher in sodium, which helps dissolve and remove such deposits. In fact there is no better food for such cases (and this includes those whose arteries have hardened because of calcium deposits, or who suffer from high blood pressure due to the narrowing of the diameter of the arteries from this cause.)

By proper use of sea vegetation in the preparation of foods, the diet may be much enriched in flavor, vitamin and mineral content, and health value, and foods may even be given a salty taste, without the use of the physiological poison known as salt, whose universal use is no excuse for its harmfulness to health. After one starts to use sea vegetation daily one commences to realize that all one's life one was literally <u>starving</u> for the trace minerals they contain, without knowing it. One then appreciates the dietetic wisdom of the Orientals who, for centuries, added sea vegetation to their diet.

There are many varieties of sea vegetation that grow off the coast of Japan, and which are eaten by the Japanese as part of their diet. Indeed, in Japan, the gathering, drying, packaging, and sales of sea vegetation is an important industry; and many varieties, neatly packed in cellophane, are exported to this country, where they are purchased chiefly by the Japanese population, Americans having not yet awakened to realize the immense nutritional value of this true Organic Super Food. However, recently, two American nutritionists (West and the writer) have made a special study of the nutritional value and possibilities of imported Japanese sea vegetation, and have commenced to recommend their dietary use as well as establish their distribution. Their experience has convinced them that not only can imported sea vegetation replace artificial vitamins and minerals, but are vastly superior to them, since they supply these substances in organic form and in natural combination with each other and with rare trace minerals found only in the ocean, on which optimal utilization of vitamins depends.

Besides serving to season foods by supplying organic sodium chloride to replace common salt and besides enriching them with vitamins and trace minerals, sea plants are also valuable for building up the body's alkali reserve, which is its greatest protection against disease and the growth of pathogenic bacteria. Sodium is an important constituent of the alkali reserve, helping in the neutralization and elimination of carbonic acid in the form of carbon dioxide, which is given off by the lungs. However, this sodium must be supplied in organic form, as provided by sea vegetation, since, when inorganic sodium chloride is ingested, rather than fortify the alkali reserve, it lowers it, and, by robbing the body of calcium, predisposes to acidosis and its after-effects, such as sinus and catarrhal conditions, colds, and such acid conditions as rheumatism. Since proteins, fats, sugars and starches all form acid products of metabolism and constantly tend to lower the alkali reserve, an alkaline blood stream is the surest guarantee of health; and sea plants help to maintain the normal alkalinity of the blood, which is the foundation of resistance to disease.

In general, sea vegetation averages 10 to 20 times more total minerals than any land-grown food. Exclusive of adhering crude sea salt (which, as already pointed out, is undesirable and should be carefully washed off before using), sea vegetation contains an average of 15% to 40% total food minerals, whereas the total mineral content of land vegetation on an ash basis averages 1% to 2%. These facts would indicate the necessity to augment the daily diet with sea vegetation to help insure a sufficient intake of organic minerals and vitamins, in quality and variety that synthetic products can never supply. Oriental races which use various types of sea vegetation as food are remarkably free from such diseases as cancer, diabetes, etc., which their mineral-and vitamin-rich diet helps them ward against.

Trace Mineral Deficiency and Disease

Dr. Charles Northen, an Alabama physician specializing in stomach disorders, came to the conclusion that most modern diseases are due to the fact that soils, and the foods they produce, fail to contain the minerals they should have, especially the trace minerals. He found that the basic causes of insect pests attacking crops was a deficiency of trace minerals. Dr. Albrecht has experimentally proven this by planting parallel rows of plants, one with and the other without trace minerals added to the soil. The plants that received the trace minerals remained immune to insect pests, while the others were attacked. Seeking a source of trace minerals to replenish exhausted soils, and thereby grow mineralized foods capable of supporting optimal health of humans, Dr. Northen found this in certain phosphate deposits in Florida which were formed through the decomposition of prehistoric marine life. This was a phosphatic clay known as colloidal phosphate. Analysis showed it to contain over twenty different trace minerals of marine origin. Addition of colloidal phosphate to the soil replaced the minerals that have been washed into the sea since ancient times, with the result that plants grew healthier, were resistant to insect pests; and humans who were fed such mineralized and vitaminized foods became free from diseases from which they previously suffered when on diets composed of foods grown on mineral-deficient soil.

Savage in Kentucky performed similar experiments, using various powdered rocks for mineralizing the soil and thus producing foods exceptionally high in mineral and vitamin content, which he considered the true cure for the ills that afflict humanity. Many sick people, hearing of Savage's work, came to his "Mineralized Gardens," camping nearby in order to regain health by living on his mineral-rich Super Foods. Savage developed his theory of rebuilding health through soil remineralization by observing that the finest horses come from his state of Kentucky, where they feed on grass grown on soil rich in decomposed rock minerals. By mineralizing the soil of his experimental farm with powdered rocks containing an abundance of trace minerals, and then feeding sick people on the mineralized foods thus produced, he was able to restore them to health. His theory was that by restoring to the soil and to plants the trace minerals they lack, and by feeding animals and humans on a diet so enriched with trace minerals, it should be possible not only to bring them to a state of perfect health, but also to regenerate them, so that they may regain the lost biological superiority of their ancestors who fed on the mineral-rich products of prehistoric soil, and thus to bring about a state of "Super Health", and to develop a Super Race, both among different animal species and among humans. The secret of achieving such biological regeneration, Savage claimed, consisted in remineralizing the soil with all the trace minerals it should contain and which were present in prehistoric soils. Addition to the soil of colloidal phosphate, a prehistoric marine deposit rich in readily available, soluble trace minerals, is one of the best way to achieve this end, as Dr. Northen has pointed out.

Dr. Northen, like Savage, maintained that a basic cause of disease is trace mineral deficiency, and that, if this is so, the only true cure of disease is to replace the missing trace minerals, in foods. There are two ways to do this: (1) to enrich foods with trace minerals from sea vegetation, thereby returning to them the elements that were washed from the soil and poured into the sea, where these sea plants gathered them and brought them back to us, (2) remineralizing the soil by addition of trace-mineral-containing powdered rocks, such as colloidal phosphate, granite (a rich source of trace minerals), etc., thereby producing foods that contain them.

Dr. Northen demonstrated that trace mineral deficiency not only causes disease among humans, but plant diseases and insect pests. He proved this latter point by growing two intertwined tomato plants, each growing in a different flower pot and fertilized differently, one being given colloidal phosphate and the other not. The plant that failed to receive the trace minerals of colloidal phosphate was attacked by pests, whereas the intertwined plant that received them was immune. This indicated that insects are scavengers that attack weakened and mineral-deficient plant tissues, but not healthy, mineralized ones. It is the same as regards bacteria in reference to the human body. The organism that is abundantly supplied with trace minerals, as a result of consuming foods grown in soil rich in them, or due to adding sea vegetation to the diet, will have optimal resistance to disease. It will not be apt to fall prey to the ravages of bacteria.

One reason why use of chemical fertilizers has led to increased prevalence of insect pests and the need for spraying (which practice was almost unknown, nor was it necessary, before chemical fertilizers were first used) is that such strong chemicals, due to their higher solubility, interfere with the plant's capacity to take up minerals, including trace minerals, from the soil, with the result that it becomes mineral-deficient. Also by growing at a faster rate, due to the forcing influence of such fertilizers, the plant fails to take up from the soil all the minerals it otherwise would do during a longer and slower growth. More chemical fertilizers, mean more insect pests, and more spraying - each of these evils following as a natural consequence of the other. And we may add, more diseases among plants, animals and humans.

Nutritional Value of Sea Vegetation

Sea vegetation is valuable because of its richness in iron, as well as in copper, manganese and cobalt, which act in conjunction with iron in hemoglobin formation. Dulse, or Irish sea lettuce, with its dark red color, is an excellent source of iron, better than liver. Bunge, the eminent biochemist, has pointed out that iron, to be effective for red blood cell formation, should be in organic form (as provided by sea vegetation), whereas inorganic iron, as provided by iron salts or mineral water, is harmful to the liver and other organs; and the body cannot use it. Prof. Sherman has also pointed out the superiority of organic over inorganic iron for hemoglobin regeneration.

Okra has been recommended as a desirable dietary supplement for sufferers from stomach and intestinal ulcers due to its natural mucilaginous properties as well as calcium content. However, certain varieties of sea vegetation possess much greater mucilaginous properties than okra, as well as more calcium, besides being richer in all essential minerals than okra, or any other land-grown vegetable.

In 1933, Meyer, Seidman and Necheles published a report in the *Illinois Medical Journal* concerning the favorable effects of the mucilaginous substance exuded by certain sea plants in cases of constipation and peptic ulcers. Mathieu writes: "In cases of gastric ulcer accompanied by constipation, this substance (i.e., mucin, or the mucilagious substance of sea plants) has produced excellent results. It even seems to have a soothing effect on stomach pains." In this respect mucin surpasses even okrin, the mucilaginous substance of okra.

West, an authority on sea vegetation, whose book we have mentioned above, objects to the use of powdered sea plants on the market, such as powdered kelp and dulse, because they contain sea salt, which has not been removed by washing before powdering, and which he considers harmful, as is all inorganic sodium chloride. He recommends instead imported Japanese sea vegetation, whose adhering sea salt can be removed by washing before using. In his book he cites the following case that has come under his observation, showing the superiority of the organic sodium chloride of sea vegetation over common salt, an inorganic chemical. Mrs. Ida H$_u$ghes of Baltimore, Md. was a chronic invalid at the age of 75, suffering from incurable arthritis. Her high blood-pressure and swollen limbs made it necessary for her to use crutches. While both of these conditions were aggravated by the use of inorganic sodium chloride, or common salt, it seemed that the organic sodium chloride of sea vegetation, as well as the other organic minerals it contains, helped her to overcome her conditions. Under the direction of her physician, she added sea vegetation to her diet, with the result that, within a year, her pains were gradually relieved, her swelling disappeared and she no longer had need for crutches. At the age of 85, she was able to run up and down a flight of stairs without panting for breath.

Dr. Frederick M. Allen, in the Journal of the American Medical Association, reports valuable effects in diabetes by use of Myrtillin, a substance found in the leaves of certain members of the myrtle family, in the dried leaves of the blueberry plant and in all sea plant leaves. It seems to aid carbohydrate metabolism and to prevent hypoglycemia. For many years blueberry leaf tea was used by the Alpine peasantry for diabetes. Dr. Richard L. Wagner of the University of Vienna subjected blueberry tea to clinical tests in diabetes and found that it tended to reduce or abolish glucosuria. It was not sure whether this was due to its myrtillin content or some associated vitamin. This would indicate that use of sea plants may be valuable for diabetes.

A well known Boston physician, enjoying an extensive medical practice, put a patient suffering from complete paralysis and grey hair on an alkaline diet including sea vegetation. According to the doctor's report, cited by West in his book above mentioned, after fifteen months the man returned to work and "during recovery his hair returned form very white color to a black shade." This change in hair color may or may not be due to the presence of the so-called anti-grey-hair vitamins in sea vegetation. However, according to a news item released by Dr. Wm. P. Brady, which appeared in a New England newspaper on June 6, 1941, it would appear that the retarded greying of the hair among Orientals may be due to the dried sea greens that they consume daily as part of their diet. West claims to have on record a number of similar reports, indicating that certain varieties of imported sea vegetation contain yet unknown nutrients (undoubtedly trace minerals) which help restore grey hair to its natural color.

Sea vegetation is rich in vitamin A, and is valuable as a dependable source of vitamin D, which tends to be lacking in most vegetable foods. The vegetarian, who tends to lack this vitamin, especially during the winter time, when he does not receive sufficient ultra-violet rays from the sun, will do well to add sea vegetation to his diet to insure a sufficient supply of this vitamin.

Sea vegetation is also a rich source of the anti-hemorrhagic vitamin K. It is also a good source of the anti-sterility vitamin E, which may be one reason for the well known fertility of Oriental races which use sea plants abundantly.

In recent times much attention was given to rose hips as a source of vitamin C, in place of citrus fruits. However, sea vegetation also supplies abundant vitamin C, lack of which is associated with chronic nasal sinusitis, rheumatoid arthritis and rheumatic fever in children. Sea plants are also rich in vitamin B complex, providing riboflavin, pyridoxine, panthothenic acid, niacin and thiamin.

In short, sea vegetation is a superior, and often a super-abundant, source of ALL essential vitamins and minerals, both major and trace minerals, both known and unknown. Their immense potential value as sources of natural vitamins and organic minerals should therefore be given much more careful attention by progressive nutritionists.

Chapter Seven

SEEDS AS SUPER SOURCES OF NUTRITION

Providing Complete Proteins, Natural Vitamins, Organic Minerals, Lecithin and Unsaturated Fatty Acids

In the seed of the plant, Nature has stored away a complete supply of nutrients - including proteins, fats, vitamins, minerals, enzymes, etc.- necessary to support the life and growth of the young seedling before it is able to secure nourishment from its environment. For this reason, seeds contain a unique combination of organically combined minerals and vitamins, in association with proteins, phospolipins and other substances necessary for the well-being and reproduction of living cells, whether of plant, animal or man - a combination which no chemist can imitate.

Seeds in the Diet of Different Races

Seeds are Nature's Supreme Pluri-Vitamin and Mineral Foods; and millions of people in various parts of the world have, since time immemorial, instinctively realized this fact by incorporating seeds as a fundamental part of their diet. Two and a half thousand years ago, the great Greek philosopher Pythagoras, who was the first scientific nutritionist in history, highly recommended the nutritional value of seeds, particularly millet and sesame seeds. Since this time, and probably before, these foods were in common use among peoples of the Near East and in Asia. Hemp seeds have also been widely used for food purposes - in India, Turkey and elsewhere. In Southeastern Europe a preferred vegetable oil is made from these seeds. In Russia, toasted sunflower seeds and virgin sunflower seed oil have always been the favorite of the peasantry, probably because sunflowers grow well in cold climates. In China, sesame and sunflower seeds are both popular. In India, sesame seeds are ground into a meal, as they also are in Japan, and are used in cooking as a source of fat and protein. Hemp seed is popular in India and is often preferred to sesame seed because of its more pronounced flavor, which is somewhat aromatic. Throughout Turkey, Lebanon, Syria, Armenia and other countries of the Near East, sesame seeds occupy an important place in the diet, as a basic source of fat and protein. They are most commonly used in the form of virgin sesame seed oil and "Tahini", a thick cream made from crushed sesame seeds, which largely replace cholesterol-containing butter, lard and other animal fats in the diet of the people of the Near East. Toasted squash and pumpkin seeds are also popular in many parts of the world, especially in Turkey, Syria, etc. In Russia pumpkin seeds are widely used, together with sunflower seeds; and in Mexico and Guatemala, a high-fat squash seed known as pepitoria is in great demand by the Indians, who shell it by hand and sell the kernels to each other by the ounce or pound in their markets. This seed is very nutritious, and one of the most healthful and digestible of all seeds; and for the Maya Indians, who used it since time immemorial, it provided an economical and healthful source of protein and fat in their diet, easier to secure from nature than animal foods, which may be one reason why this race has lived on a more or less vegetarian diet. (The avocado, which grows so abundantly in both the lowlands and highlands of Guatemala, home of the Mayas, and which provides a perfect substitute for meat, eggs and dairy products, also contributed to their being able to maintain themselves so successfully without animal foods.) The pepitoria kernel, as used by the Indians, is generally used by first toasting over a hot earthenware pan, whereupon it swells like popcorn, and becomes crisp. It is then often crushed by stone into a meal and added to various foods. Melon seeds are also used by the Guatemalan Indians and also in the Near East. They are generally soaked, ground and prepared into a milk which bears remarkable resemblence to cow's milk, souring in the same manner, after which it may be made into a cheese. (Similar dairy product substitutes may be made from sesame seeds, alone or in combination with coconut milk.)

While the so-called "backward" races of various parts of the world possess the dietetic wisdom to incorporate seeds in their diet, which supply them with a wealth of nutritional essentials, the American people, who are supposed to be the most advanced in civilization, seem to be in almost complete ignorance of the immense nutritional value of seeds, which occupy only an insignificant part of the American diet - except for caraway seeds used in rye bread and sesame and poppy seeds used in cakes. In place of seeds as a source of natural vitamins, artificial synthetic products are used, which are much inferior in value.

Rodale Starts Seed-Eating Movement in America

About a decade ago, J.I. Rodale, father of the organic gardening and farming movement in America, developed an interest in the sunflower seed as a possible dietary supplement, and after studying it for some time and experimenting with it in his own diet and in that of his friends, he published a pamphlet, "Sunflower Seeds the Miracle Food", in which he described the various nutritional qualities of this seed, including its capacity to end the gum bleeding of pyorrhea, which he has observed in several cases. He also extolled the nutritional virtues of the sunflower seed as a source of major and trace minerals, vitamins, proteins, etc.

Soon sunflower-seed-eating become a dietary fad which spread from coast to coast, and from a formerly neglected seed, called "polly seed" because used chiefly for feeding parrots, sunflower seeds became part of the diet of increasing numbers of progressive health-seekers; and the plantings of sunflower seeds increased manyfold to meet this new demand. But what was new in America, as was the case when the soy bean was first introduced, was old in other parts of the world, where sunflower seeds were eaten for centuries, as by the Russians and Chinese.

In 1949, soon after preparing the original draft of the book "How To Eat Safely in a Poisoned World", in which he mentioned both sunflower and sesame seeds, the writer developed an interest in the sesame seed, which was then as unknown in America as the sunflower seed was before Rodale popularized it. He then encouraged a friend who was starting a new health food mail order business to advertise sesame seeds and sesame seed products, and commence their distribution, while he published a number of articles on the nutritional value of sesame seeds in the magazines Nature's Path and Organic Gardening (writing under a pen name, as is his custom). He then sent some samples of sesame seed products to its editor, Mr. Rodale, to test in his diet; and the latter wrote back admitting that he believed that the sesame seed had even greater possibilities as a new food for America than the sunflower seed, due to its greater nutritional versatility. Rodale's prediction was later fulfilled, for the sesame seed was soon enthusiastically taken up by progressive dietetians everywhere, who soon appreciated its wonderful dietary qualities as a super source of highly digestible, non-acid-forming, purin-free complete proteins, lecithin, vitamins in abundance and organically combined calcium, iron and other minerals. And in addition, sesame seed products have a most delicious flavor. New producers and distributors of sesame seed products then sprang up all over the country; and these products became good sellers in health food stores from coast to coast.

After he started the sesame seed on its nutritional career in America, the writer, during a trip to Central America, came across another seed that interested him, and which he also introduced into this country as a new food. It is the peritoria squash seed, an ancient food of the Maya Indians, which is still eaten today, and which they prefer to both sunflower and sesame seeds, as the writer himself did after he tried it in his diet.

Later the writer developed an interest in other seeds, such as hemp seeds, pumpkin seeds and Turkish squash seeds, all of which he found to possess interesting and valuable nutritional possibilities. (Organic Food Research Associates, 215 Sixth St., Lorain, Ohio is now distributing a large number of products made from hemp seeds, as well as sesame and sunflower seeds.) As for the pumpkin seed, due to its larger size and softer composition, when toasted, it is most deliciously crunchy and digestible, and is well worthy of dietary use, though previously its use was largely medicinal (i.e., raw pumpkin seeds were eaten as worm expellers). Another seed that the writer found used among the Maya Indians is the canteloupe seed, from which is made substitute for cow's milk (also for other milk derivatives as clabber and cheese), that bears remarkable resemblence to cow's products in all respects. Watermelon seeds are the one seed for which he found no dietary use, though their medicinal value as a source of substance that has proven extremely valuable in the treatment of kidney diseases has been widely recognized.

Seeds as Sources of Nutritionally Essential Unsaturated Fatty Acids
(Vitamin F)

Far too little interest has been given by nutritionists to vitamin F and its importance for health. For some mysterious reason, this vitamin has been neglected, while others have been given almost exclusive attention. Perhaps one reason for this is that sources of vitamin F are cheap, and that it cannot be synthetically produced - hence bringing much smaller profits to vitamin manufacturers than the snythetic vitamins. (Vitamin F, or the unsaturated fatty acids, lenoleic and lenolenic, is present in all seeds, large amounts being contained in flaxseed and linseed oil, a comparatively inexpensive oil.)

A little over twenty years ago, Burr and Burr first showed that vitamin F was essential in nutrition, and that when it was lacking in the diet, animals failed in health. The skin, nervous system and endocrine glands (especially the prostate gland) seem to depend on its presence and to suffer from its lack. Biochemists are now agreed that vitamin F is an indispensable ingredient of the diet, and is of the nature of an unsaturated fatty acid, being an isomer of linoleic and linolenic acids, present in linseed oil as well as in most other seeds, including sesame seeds. Summarizing the known nutritional importance of unsaturated fatty acids, or vitamin F, in the diet, McCollum and Becker say; " A diet containing everything else which is essential, but lacking linoleic acid will fail to maintain life. Linoleic acid (vitamin F) must therefore be provided in the food."

Seeds appear to be the most reliable source of vitamin F in nature, in fact the <u>only</u> reliable source, since this vitamin is not present to any appreciable extent in any other food except seeds and their raw, unrefined oils. Nor can it be synthetically produced, which fact, as already indicated, explains why pharmaceutical concerns financing vitamin research and dispensing vitamins developed little interest in it, so that it became the black sheep of the vitamin family. Since pharmaceutical concerns are interested only in what they can make profit on, and since the best source of vitamin F is raw linseed oil, they saw no economic future for them to popularize and sell this vitamin, as they did others which were really no more important or essential for health. The result was that large numbers of people, knowing little or nothing about the existence of vitamin F and its importance in their diet, neglected to obtain sufficient to meet their requirements, so that lack of vitamin F became a widespread, though unrecognized, dietary deficiency, affecting large numbers of people living on modern refined foods, such as refined cereals and vegetable oils, whose vitamin F had been removed.

The richest natural source of vitamin F is cold-pressed raw, unrefined oils as extracted from seeds, such as linseed oil, etc. Though used in this country chiefly for the manufacture of paints, linseed oil, or the oil pressed from flax seeds, has been widely used in Central Europe as an edible oil; and while Americans, unaccustomed to it, might dislike its paint-like taste (due more to psychological association than to anything else), as a matter of fact, linseed oil, when pure and unrefined, is one of the most nutritious dietary sources of fat known, being very rich in unsaturated fatty acids (vitamin F) and other fat-soluble vitamins.

Since raw, virgin oils are unstable and tend to become rancid, to create a more stable and marketable product, they are generally refined. The refining process removes their vital elements that are responsible for their deterioration; and this involves the removal of their vitamins, sterols, unsaturated fatty acids and phosphatides, including lecithin. The resulting product is generally tasteless, and lacking the balancing factors which have been removed, tends to be much more acid-forming than raw or virgin oils. (However, it should be noted that most so-called virgin olive oils on the market have been refined to some extent to stabilize them, differing from the thick, dark oil as pressed from the olive. Such an oil is now imported from Turkey, but is not popular here, since people are accustomed to the clarified, refined type of virgin olive oil.)

Not only vegetable oils, but oleomargarines are also refined, the refining process removing the vitamin A, E and F content of the original oils from which they are made, which has led to the addition of vitamin A to "enrich" them with some of the vitamins they have been deprived of.

However, vitamin F, the most neglected of all vitamins, and the one that is most lacking in the American diet, is not put back. (A very excellent oleomargarine and butter substitute, which looks and tastes much like cow's butter, and which is rich in vitamin F and other fat-soluble vitamins absent from most margarines, as well as in lecithin, is now being distributed by Organic Food Research Associates, 215 Sixth St., Lorain, Ohio. It is known as "soya lecithin butter". This product is valuable for all who suffer vitamin F deficiency, to use in place of ordinary butter, which has little or none of this vitamin.)

To enrich the diet with vitamin F, it is best to use cold-pressed raw, virgin vegetable oils, several of which are now on the market, including virgin sesame seed oil, virgin sunflower seed oil, Turkish unrefined virgin oil of olives, and virgin soybean oil. Also, by using sesame seeds and sunflower seeds and their products, which are rich in unsaturated fatty acids, this vitamin may be secured. Squash seeds, pumpkin seeds, flax seeds and hempseeds are all good sources of this vitamin. Hempseed oil, which is a highly nutritious oil used in Southeastern Europe, where it is preferred to other vegetable oils, is an excellent source of vitamin F, as is also poppy seed oil. It is strange that while these superior vitamin-rich oils are not used to any extent by the American people, the most inferior oil, cottonseed oil, is the one most commonly sold as an edible oil. It is well known that the cottonseed contains a toxic substance and is the worst of all seeds as a human food. A very excellent virgin soybean oil is now on the market, rich in lecithin (of which it contains about 2%) and unsaturated fatty acids (vitamin F) and containing sterols (tocopherol, or vitamin E) and other soya phosphatides, including cephalin, choline, inositol and lipositol.

Besides being found in seeds, vitamin F is present in the oil of grains, especially in corn, whose fat contains considerable vitamin F and lecithin, more so than other less fatty grains, though millet, which is botanically related to corn, shares this quality to some extent, which may be indicated by the fact that both millet and corn have the characteristic yellow color of foods rich in phosphorus-rich fats (lecithin and other phosphatides), as is the case with egg yolk. Since most grains, like vegetable oils, are today refined, with the result that their vitamin F and lecithin content is removed, we can understand why most people today suffer a lack of these nutritional essentials, so important for the health, vigor and well-being of the endocrine glands and the central nervous system. In addition to the modern widespread use of nerve poisons, as tobacco, coffee, etc. and of vegetables and fruits containing toxic insecticide residues, the lack of these nerve and brain nutrients in lecithin-poor refined modern foods must play a role in the increase of nervous and mental diseases in recent times.

Do You Suffer From Symptoms of Vitamin F Deficiency?

Symptoms suggesting vitamin F deficiency are apparently more prevalent among humans than was heretofore realized. Skin conditions and allergies are now known to be due to lack of this vitamin, since unsaturated fatty acids are known to be markedly deficient in the blood serum during the active phase of eczema. There are reports of clinical cure of eczema by administration of oils rich in linoleic acid.

There is some evidence that lack of vitamin F may cause prostate disorders. According to a report issued by the Lee Institute of Nutritional Research, addition of unsaturated fatty acids to the diet of prostate sufferers brought remarkable improvement.

Widespread Vitamin F Deficiency: Why Vitamin F has been neglected by nutritionists

Both nutritionally essential unsaturated fatty acids and lecithin have been greatly neglected, not only by research financed by pharmaceutical corporations which saw little profit in their sale - but also by modern nutritionists, whose views and theories are, to a large extent, greatly influenced and even dominated by such financed research. Since the pharmaceutical interests and their paid research workers disregarded lecithin and vitamin F, the nutritionists followed suit anddid the same, in spite of the fact that these two nutritional essentials, more than any others, tend to be lacking in the American diet, with the result that large numbers of people suffer from their deficiency. (According to certain research workers, the common cold, so widespread among Americans, is one of the symptoms of vitamin F deficiency; dandruff is another; and eczematous skin disorders are still another. Obviously the pharmaceutical interests saw more profit in selling nostrums and patent medicines to relieve these conditions than to sell cheap vitamin-F-containing raw vegetable oils to prevent them.)

However, in Germany, where biochemistry first developed as an independent science and where it reached a high state of development before it was seriously studied in this country, the attitude of nutritionists and scientists toward lecithin and its associated unsaturated fatty acids (both of which tend to occur together in seeds and raw vegetable oils) was quite different, since German scientific research was more disinterested and not dominated by commercial interests to the extent that occurs in this country. The nutritional and therapeutic value of lecithin and its associated substances was there widely recognized and employed by the medical profession for glandular, nervous and mental conditions, and soybean lecithin products were widely sold in drug stores for this purpose, at a time when they were practically unknown in this country, and when the American medical profession, which had never given lecithin the attention it merits, were skeptical of its physiological effects and nutritional and therapeutic virtues.

Symptoms of vitamin F deficiency include; dry, rough, peeling skin, with a tendency to pigmentation, a proneness to develop sores and an ultimate eczema, falling hair, dandruff, brittle and ridged finger nails (fluted), fatiguability, distress in hot weather, susceptibility to vitamin D and sun poisoning, friability of bones (especially in the aged), constipation, hemorrhoids, renal irritation with hematuria and albuminura, glycosuria, disturbed fat metabolism evidenced by overweight or improperly distributed fat pads and many allergic symptoms, such as giant hives, susceptibility to colds, etc.

The universality of the common cold is one of the most evident symptoms of vitamin F deficiency. Drs. E.M. Boyd and W.F. McConnell conducted a research to determine whether widespread vitamin F deficiency was a cause of the common cold. They reported their findings in an article, "Essential Fatty Acids in the Relief of the Common Cold" (<u>Canadian Medical Journal</u> 37: 38 July 1937). A total of 106 young men, mostly medical students, took part in the experiment. Forty-one were subject to frequent and severe colds each winter. Sixty-five were relatively free from colds. Use of vitamin F resulted in a significant lowering of colds in 64% of those that were susceptible. The study suggested that a considerable part of the population suffers from colds as a result of unsaturated fatty acid deficiency, since the effect of the unsaturated fatty acids on the duration of each cold fell from an average of 11.2 days before treatment to an average of 2.5 days while under vitamin F therapy. This was a decrease of 78%. Ten of the men suffering from chronic nasal catarrh reported improvement. Four were greatly relieved; three noticed a worthwile improvement and three a partial one.

In 1935, Oncken reported experiments showing that the vitamin F content of the blood is reduced in mild infections such as the common head cold. They found that when unsaturated fatty acids were excluded from the diet of animals, though other fats were present, they failed to grow properly. Supplementing the deficient diet with unsaturated fatty acids brought a return to normal.

These observations indicate the importance of increasing the consumption of seeds and the unrefined oils of seeds to supply the essential unsaturated fatty acids (vitamin F) which are lacking in butter, other animan fats, refined vegetable oils and oleomargarines.

Seeds as Sources of Lecithin, a Hitherto Unrecognized Nutritional Essential

In addition to unsaturated fatty acids, seeds are also valuable as a source of lecithin, a phosphorized nerve and brain fat of which seeds are one of the best sources. There is considerable evidence that lecithin, though much neglected by nutritionists in the past, is a dietary essential that may be ranked with proteins, fats and carbohydrates in importance. It is an essential constituent of the nuclei of all cells, controlling the basic processes of oxidation and cell metabolism. Without lecithin, there could be no life. And as in the case of the unsaturated fatty acids, lecithin tends to be lacking in the modern diet; and seeds are its best source. It is almost entirely absent from modern refined foods, though present in grains and vegetable oils prior to refining. It is closely associated with the unsaturated fatty acids and sterols (including tocopherol, or vitamin E). Soya lecithin, as extracted from raw soybean oil, is always found in associated soya phosphatides, as cephalin, choline, inositol and lipositol. While choline and inositol have been given more attention and their nutritional value recognized as factors of the vitamin B complex, there is reason to believe that all these substances, including cephalin, a brain fat, play an important and essential role in nutrition. Biotin, another vitamin B factor, has been found in association with the lecithin of seeds and soy beans.

Not much is known about the functions of the other phosphatides associated with lecithin, such as cephalin, inositol and choline, whose physiological roles in animal and human nutrition are not well known or understood.

The exact requirements for inositol and choline are not well defined, though they are thought to be high. There is every reason to believe that the other soya phosphatides associated with lecithin have a complementary, and important, physiological function, and that the beneficial effects of adding lecithin to the diet is due partly to these associated phosphatides. We must also remember that soybean lecithin yields about 3% organically combined phosphorus, which is almost entirely available for animal and human nutrition. The phosphorus in lecithin, unlike that in phtin, is readily available for bone formation.

Foods rich in lecithin are: eggs, legumes, seeds, corn, millet, etc. But while eggs are rich in lecithin, they are also rich in cholesterol, which is harmful. Also the lecithin of egg yolk tends to quickly decompose to form choline, which reduces to neurine, a nerve irritant. When one eats whole eggs to obtain lecithin, one takes in the albumen of the white of the egg, which tends to strain the kidneys, since it represents an excess of protein which the adult body cannot use, and which must be eliminated through the kidneys. Also eggs tend to rapidly undergo intestinal putrefaction and are constipating. They also tend to be infected with disease germs. The chicken is a filthy creature, which eats bugs, insects, worms, etc. when it has the opportunity; and under such conditions, these are the raw materials from which eggs are made.

Sesame seeds are good sources of lecithin, which they provide in a balanced alkaline form, in association with minerals. Use of sesame seed products for lecithin is to be highly recommended.

Nutritionists in the past have considered fats merely as hydrocarbons and replacable by carbohydrates, since both were considered valuable only as sources of carbon, which, when oxidized, changes to carbonic acid and carbon dioxide, or is deposited as fat. Later it was shown that certain fats were bearers of fat-soluble vitamins (A, D, E and F), and so were important aside from their carbon content, and were not replacable by carbohydrates. And still later, nutritional research has ascertained that certain fats also contain other substances of high physiological value - lecithin and related phosphatides, which are important for the endocrine glands, nervous system and red blood cells. These phosphorus-rich fats are present chiefly in the germ of grains and in seeds, and tend to be absent from modern refined foods. This is why it is important to include in the diet seeds or some other source of lecithin to supply this nutritional essential, which not only is lacking in most modern foods, but whatever little is present is often withdrawn and lost by present methods of food preparation, especially the use of aluminum utensils in the cooking of foods, since it has been shown that aluminum, dissolved from the walls of such utensils and taken up by foods, combines with the organic phosphorus of lecithin, which is taken away from the spinal cord and central nervous system, thus creating a deficiency or augmenting a deficiency which may have previously existed. Bleaching and preservative chemicals added to white and whole wheat flour seem to have a similar effect, which partly explains their injurious effect on the nervous system.

Physiological Function of Lecithin

Lecithin was first discovered by Gobley in 1846. Through his labors and those of subsequent investigators, the presence of this substance was recognized in a great variety of animal and vegetable organisms and especially in the eggs of birds, fish roe, brain substance, yeast, etc. It is now recognized as a constitutent of every animal and vegetable cell - this universality of distributing indicating its indispensability to life.

Phosphorus and lecithin are essential constituents of the nuclei of all cells; and without lecithin life in the cell, which depends on the basic processes of metabolism and oxidation, which lecithin governs, is impossible. The presence of lecithin in the cell protects it against the adverse effects of cholesterol, which, when present in excess, tends to diminish the permeability of the cell wall. For this reason, under conditions of lecithin deficiency and cholesterol excess, cellular overnutrition and suboxidation result, which lay the groundwork for the development of cancer.

Just as lecithin is a dominating substance which directs cell life and metabolism, being present in its nucleus, so in the human body, lecithin, in combination with cephalin, is present largely in the brain, and is a primary constituent of the myelin sheath of the nerves, which it acts as an oil whose burning supports the electrical fire of nerve activity. Lecithin is also a chief constituent of those fatty organs, which direct the functioning of the other organs of the body, the endocrine glands; and there is evidence that it is needed for their normal activity and performance of their hormone functions.

There is more lecithin in the grey matter of the brain, the seat of the intellectual processes, than in the white matter, which consists chiefly of connective fibers; and the importance of lecithin for brain functioning is demonstrated by the fact that while the normal brain contains about 28% lecithin, that of the insane was found to contain only 14%. Obviously deficiency of lecithin must play some role in the origin of insanity, which is indicated by the observation of German neurologists and psychiatrists concerning the beneficial effect of lecithin in nervous and mental conditions.

Other vital organs, as the heart, liver and kidneys, are also rich in lecithin, which is also abundant in the gonads and the reproductive cells, lack of lecithin being a factor in the origin of sterility. This is proven by the fact that wheat germ oil, one of the richest sources of the anti-sterility vitamin E, is very rich in lecithin, and that pure tocopherol fails to have the anti-sterility effect of wheat germ oil containing tocopherols in combination with lecithin, which would indicate that much of the effect of wheat germ oil in preventing and curing sterility is due to its lecithin content.

Formerly the brain and spinal cord of animals was used as a source of lecithin for therapeutic purposes, but more recently the soy bean has become the chief commercial source. Soybean lecithin has been widely used as a dietary supplement and as an additive to vitamins, in view of its capacity to increase the assimilation and utilization of certain vitamins, especially vitamin A.

Due to its emulsifying property, soybean lecithin has found commercial use in the manufacture of oleomargarines, helping to keep their oils in emulsion, and in the making of chocolate. Due to its emulsifying properties, lecithin has been found to aid fat metabolism, promoting better absorption of fatty substances in the intestines. (Fats must be emulsified in order to be properly assimilated; and lecithin brings them into emulsion. For this reason lecithin aids in the intestinal absorption of certain fat-soluble vitamins, as vitamin A. It also helps in the conversion of carotene into vitamin A in the body. This emulsifying property of lecithin explains why virgin oils, rich in lecithin, are more digestible than refined oils, whose lecithin has been removed, since the fats of the latter, being in a non-emulsified form tend to be improperly assimilated and form free fatty acids. For this reason refined vegetable oils are more acid-forming than unrefined virgin oils containing lecithin.)

Addition of lecithin to vitamin A has been found to lead to greater liver storage of this vitaman, and to greater gain in weight of the young growing organism. Lecithin also increases the efficiency of vitamin E provided by wheat germ oil (one of the richest sources of lecithin), and this is why pure tocopherol without lecithin is not as effective as wheat germ oil with it.

Lecithin, through the choline it yields, has a beneficial effect on liver function and well-being. It aids in the metabolism of fats and carbohydrates in the liver, and prevents fatty accumulations in this organ, correcting disturbances of fat metabolism. Fats are transformed in the liver into lecithin, and dietary lecithin promotes this process by supplying necessary building stones.

An important property of lecithin is to counteract the deposit of cholesterol in the arteries, causing them to harden. Lecithin keeps cholesterol in solution and thus tends to prevent hardening of the arteries, as well as the formation of gall stones. One of the ailments traced to cholesterol deposits is cancer.

A hitherto unrecognized dietary factor has been found in the lecithin of seeds and soy beans, provided it has not been overheated during its extraction. It is also present in raw foods, and is sensitive to heat, being destroyed in cooking and processing operations. Certain skin diseases have been attributed to a lack of this dietary factor. By supplying it, lecithin is believed to have a protective effect on certain eczemas of nutritional origin. This would indicate that persons who live mostly on cooked foods and who avoid raw vegetables and fruits due to spray residues, would do well to add seeds to their diet to supply this essential dietary otherwise supplied by raw vegetables and fruits.

Is Lecithin a Nervo and Brain Nutrient?

Although the search for an ideal native combination of organized phosphorus dates back for decades, and the introduction of animal extracts into medicine called attention to the fact that lecithin was present in these substances, the therapeutic use of the latter perse, and for specific indications, is due directly to experiments made by Danilewski in 1895.

This physiologist found that young animals fed with lecithin grew more rapidly and exhibited a larger amount of brain substance than controls. The first change induced appeared to consist of a great increase in the number of red blood corpuscles, followed by an increase of appetite, which often became voracious. In healthy adult human beings, nutrition and brain power appear to be augmented, and in the aged, vitality and recuperative power increased. These observations of the effects of lecithin made by Danilewski and his pupils have been abundantly repeated and amplified in all parts of the world, and have thus been corroborated. Professor W. Koch has devoted much time to the study of lecithin from the chemical side, and also Shinkishi Hatsi, experimenting with some of Koch's product.

Lecithin was introduced into therapeutics immediately after the publication of Danilewski's experiments. One of the first to recognize its great importance was Prof. A. Robin of Paris. The literature on lecithin has now become voluminous. Without exception, there is a consensus of opinion concerning the favorable estimate of lecithin as an important contribution to practical medicine.

Furst (Therap. Monatsch. Aug. 1903) deals almost wholly with the employment of lecithin in cerebral exhaustion. The cerebral cortex, the grey matter in general, is twice as rich in lecithin as is the white nervous matter, and the nervous centers in general depend for the highest performance of their functions on lecithin, and must obtain it from the lecithin of the blood. Alos, studies have shown that while the brain of the insane contains about half as much lecithin as the normal brain, indicating that lecithin deficiency may be an important cause of insanity. The action of anesthetics and alcohol on the brain seems to depend to some extent on their capacity to dissolve its lecithin. It follows, therefore, that certain classes of individuals are more likely than others to be deprived of their normal quota of this substance; thus the anemic and debilitated subject, the brain worker and the growing child might suffer alike from an insufficient supply of lecithin; the first named because of the general impoverishment of the blood, the second because of the increased utilization of lecithin (by the brain), and the third because of the rapid development of the cerebral cortex, which (dried) is said to contain nearly eighteen per cent of this constituent.

Believing that lecithin does its good largely by its direct action upon the cerebral cortex, Furst employed it in all the cases where, from this point of view, it is indicated, and with excellent results. What is true of the brain alone should be true of the nervous system as a whole. Naturally most cases of neurasthenia belong under cerebral exhaustion, but whenever this condition is dependent upon insufficiency of the nerve-centers in the base of the brain, medulla, spinal cord, etc., we may look to lecithin to confer a corresponding degree of improvement. Again, whenever neurasthenia is a symptom of general chronic affections, such as consumption or diabetes, the patient's sufferings are much diminished by the action of lecithin upon the nervous system.

A study of the chemical changes in nerve tissue which are affected by organic disease appears to show that lecithin is decomposed whenever there is structural alteration, some of its derivatives (choline, etc.) escaping into the blood or cerebro-spinal fluid. There occurs a special waste of organic phosphorus; and if regeneration of nerve tissue were possible, it should only come about through the assimilation of lecithin. We have reason to believe that neurasthenia is an organic disease arising from lecithin deficiency in nerve tissue, and that the greatest aid in overcoming this condition is a sufficiency of lecithin in the blood. There is ground for supposing that neurasthenia is as much a lecithin deficiency disease as that beri beri is a disease of vitamin B deficiency, and that a sufficient supply of lecithin will cause it to disappear, just as a sufficient supply of vitamin B will cause the other nerve disease, beri beri, to end. (It is interesting to note that substances that are richest in natural vitamin B complex, such as brewer's yeast, corn germ, wheat germ, soybeans, etc. are also rich in lecithin. Wheat germ oil, one of the richest sources of vitamin E, is also at the same time one of the richest sources of lecithin.

The simplest conception of lecithin is that of a cellular reconstituent, especially a reconstituent of nerve, brain and red blood cells. A New York physician, after adding soybean lecithin to the diet of patients with anemia, reported a rise in the red blood cell count of over 100% within a period of several weeks, which would indicate that lecithin plays an important role in the regeneration of hemoglobin. It also appears to be equally important for the regeneration of nervous tissue; a sufficient supply of lecithin is important for the restoration of weakened and depleted nerves. According to various investigators, lecithin has furnished excellent results in hysterical and sexual neurasthenia.

Just as impoverished blood needs iron, so impoverished nervous tissue needs phosphorus in the form of lecithin. But while phosphorus is an important constituent of lecithin, lecithin is very much more than phosphorus. It is a general "intermediary of nutrition" which promotes the assimilation of various food substances, such as fats, proteins, vitamins, etc. It is undoubtedly as a result of this property that it favors the multiplication of cell life, and leads to a rapid increase of growth and weight. It increases appetite and tissue formation. While in lowly organisms, animal and plant, this increase involves the whole organism, in highly organized mammals it appears to be restricted largely to the blood corpuscles. We may assume therefore that aside from acting as a reconstituent to tissues naturally rich in lecithin (chiefly the brain), lecithin is a powerful stimulant to general nutrition through its effect in augmenting the multiplication of the red blood cells. It is also noteworthy that lecithin belongs to the lipoids or fat-like substances that act as intermediaries of nutrition through their solvent and emulsifying power, by which substances naturally insoluble in protoplasm are incorporated therein.

According to Kossel, one of the greatest authorities on organically combined phosphorus, lecithin promotes the excretion of uric acid as a result of leucocytosis. This property should make it of great value in conditions dependent on derivative elimination of uric acid, as in rhematism, goat, etc. Lecithin is of value in the treatment of tuberculosis for more reasons than one, for not only does it promote the increase of red blood cells and all that this implies (increased nutrition), but, as stated, it is directly beneficial for the nervous exhaustion which is so often present. The use of lecithin in this affection has been introduced by

Claude and Zeky, and has been recommended by the eminent authority Bouchard. The use of egg yolk, rich in lecithin, has been widely used in this disease, but soybean, corn or seed lecithin has the advantage in that it is not liable to toxic decomposition, with resulting formation of choline and neurine (a nerve poison) as is the case with egg lecithin. Also, free use of egg yolk, while it introduces considerable lecithin, provides objectionable amounts of cholesterol, which causes hardening of the arteries, gall stones and cancer.

Besides being a primary constituent of nerve and brain tissue, lecithin is present abundantly in the endocrine glands, which degenerate and fail in their hormone-producing capacity when it is lacking. The endocrine glands, including the liver, being fatty tissues, contain more lecithin than other organs of the body, except the nervous system and brain, the pineal gland containing more lecithin than all others. European specialists have considered impotence and sterility as a lecithin deficiency of the gonads, whose secretions are very rich in lecithin; and have used lecithin preparations for the treatment of these conditions, and as a reconstituent in sexual exhaustion.

From the above, it is clear that since few foods in common use supply lecithin to any extent, except egg yolk, which has the disadvantages given, seeds and the virgin oils of seeds are of great value as a source of this valuable nutrient. For some years lecithin extracted from the soy bean has been on the market and has been widely used. However, the writer found that the lecithin of seeds, such as sesame seeds, pepitoria squash seeds, pumpkin seeds, etc. was better, since seeds supply lecithin in emulsified form, and in combination with acid-forming minerals, which is better and safer to use than factory-made concentrated extracts, though, for therapeutic use, it must be admitted that soybean lecithin has its place as a dietary supplement.

NUTRITIONAL VALUE OF SESAME SEEDS

In Oriental folklore, the phrase "Open Sesame.'" was believed to place at man's command an invisible magic power that granted him fulfillment of his dreams, opening up a new world of splendor. Probably this reverence for the tiny seed was based on the deep-seated appreciation that the peoples of the Near East had for this wonderful food, which played a basic role in their diet since time immemorial.

Strangely, in spite of its tremendous a dietary possibilities, nutritionists of the past have almost completely neglected this wonderful seed, as shown by the fact that its exact vitamin and mineral content has never been fully determined. Yet the little that is known about it would indicate that this ancient food of the human race, which is still a basic food among teeming millions in Turkey, Syria, Lebanon and other countries of the Near East, contains a wealth of nutritional essentials of highly possible value and digestibility - including complete proteins, lecithin-rich fats, vitamins and minerals. Also it has an alkaline reaction, which makes sesame seed protein and fat, which exist in combination with alkaline minerals, far superior to most other proteins and fats, which are aicd-forming and hence more difficult to digest.

The protein content of sesame seeds is about 36% which is about 50% more than that of meat and most other proteins. Experience has proven that it is one of the most easily digested of all proteins. Some sesame seed meal or cream dressing spread over foods, such as salad, cereals, vegetables or legumes, provides at the same time an abundance of high quality proteins, fats and lecithin, as well as the nutritionally essential unsaturated fatty acids (vitamin F) which most foods in common use lack.

We may list the following reasons why sesame seeds and its products, of which there are now a dozen or more on the market (sesame seed meal, butter, cream dressing, oil, etc.), should occupy an important place in your diet:

1. Because they are excellent sources of unsaturated fatty acids (vitamin F) and lecithin, both of which tend to be lacking in most modern refined diets.

2. They are good sources of vitamin E, also vitamins A, B, and C.

3. They are valuable sources of organic calcium and phosphorus for the teeth and bones, and iron for the blood.

4. They are a super source of high quality, easily digested, non-acid-forming complete proteins, containing all essential amino acids otherwise provided by the best animal proteins (meat, eggs and milk). They are better than animal proteins because, they do not tend to putrefy in the intestines or cause constipation and autointoxication, as animal proteins do. Also they are rich in alkaline minerals, which prevents their proteins from having any acid effects, and so are valuable for sufferers from acidosis. Not only do sesame seeds provide proteins of high quality and digestibility, valuable in the diet of persons who are sick, run down and who have weak digestions, but they supply nearly 50% more protein than do most animal protein foods, as meat, eggs and cheese. Also, they are free from putrefactive bacteria and disease germs, as are present in meat, eggs and milk.

5. Nature has locked in this seed a wealth of nutrients, known and unknown, so that its daily use will help protect one against dietary deficiencies, both those of which one is aware as well as those that one knows nothing about.

6. Sesame seed products are very tasty and add flavor as well as extra nutrition to other foods. Sprinkling sesame seed meal over salads, cereals, vegetables and other foods enriches them with high quality proteins, unsaturated fatty acids, lecithin and vitamins. The meal may be used in cooking in place of other acid-forming and cholesterol containing fats, as vegetable oils, oleomargarine and butter. Sesame seed meal may also be incorporated in baked products as a shortening, and is excellent added to soups, giving them a creamy richness.

Sesame seeds combine the virtues of a rich source of natural vitamins with those of a nutritious, tasty food, supplying highly digestible, non-acid-forming, nonputrefying proteins and fats. While they are richer in protein than most other proteins, including animal proteins and nuts, they are more digestible because more alkaline, most other protein foods tending to be acid-forming. Sesame seed protein is also superior to meat, egg and milk proteins in being free from cholesterol, which they contain; and cholesterol, as is known, is a cause of cancer. Sufferers from constipation and autointoxication will do well to use sesame seed products in place of animal proteins, since they do not putrefy and decay in the intestines and form toxic end-products of intestinal putrefaction, which paralyze the intestinal muscles and cause constipation and autointoxication, as animal proteins do. Those who suffer from acidosis, and the diseases that arise from this cause, as hardening of the arteries, high blood pressure, rheumatism, etc., will do well to use sesame seed protein in place of acid-forming animal proteins, as meat, eggs and cheese, and also in place of acid-forming nut proteins and uric-acid-forming legumes. (Lima beans and navy beans are highly alkaline; and so are chick peas, or garbanzos. The alkalinity of the lima bean is especially high when it is in the green state.)

Due to their high content of readily assimilable phosphorus, sesame seeds are valuable for brain workers. In addition to organic phosphorus in the form of phosphates, as present in fruits and vegetables, they contain the more highly organized fatty phosphorus compound known as lecithin, a nerve and brain fat which we have previously discussed. They provide lecithin in a balanced form, in combination with alkaline minerals, which is better than extracted soybean lecithin that has been deprived of the balancing effect of the alkaline minerals with which it was originally associated. Sesame seeds contain the whole alphabet of vitamins, known and unknown, and supply them in a natural, organic form in combination with minerals, lecithin and other phosphatides, as well as enzymes, all of which aid in the assimilation and utilization of vitamins. Therefore we can heartily recommend: Use sesame seeds and sesame seed products as a source of vitamins, in place of synthetics!

<u>Dairy Product Substitutes Made from Sesame Seeds</u>:

Sesame Seed Milk, Cream, Butter, Clabber and Cheese

From the sesame seed, by use of a liquefier with blades capable of liquefying it, dairy product substitutes may be made which provide healthful substitutes for cow's milk and its derivatives, having the advantage of being bacteria - and cholesterol - free, while at the same time providing high quality proteins, calcium, phosphorus, vitamins and minerals present in milk, besides iron, which milk lacks. Also sesame seed milk is free from putrefactive bacteria and disease germs present in milk and is not liable to transmit undulent fever, as raw milk does, while it provides abundant organic calcium, which pasteurized milk fails to do, since the pasteurization process makes the calcium of milk unavailable. Also while cow's milk is mucus-forming and constipating to adults, sesame seed milk, with its more highly alkaline reaction and freedom from putrefactive tendency, is free from this objection.

Sesame seed milk sours like cow's milk and turns into a clabber from which a cheese may be made that is more healthful than cow's cheese, and a much better source of calcium than the pasteurized cheeses on the market. Pasteurized milk and cheese, since their friendly, acidophilic bacteria have been killed by the pasteurization process, while the harmful putrefactive varieties have not, tend to rot in the intestine, causing constipation and autointoxication. Sesame seed milk, being pure and free from bacteria, on the other hand, requires no pasteurization and therefore is a much better food from the standpoint of intestinal hygiene. But even if it were possible to secure clean, disease-free raw milk, the stomach of the adult is constitutionally unable to digest its tough curd. Milk is a food intended only for a young growing organism; and no adult animal after the age of weaning will touch it. Even for infants, cow's milk, with its excessive protein and calcium content, lower lecithin content, tougher curd and greater tendency to putrefy, is not a good food. Coconut milk, or coconut-sesame seed milk, are better. We generally recommend combining sesame seed and coconut for the preparation of vegetable milk for infant feeding, since the lower protein content of coconut milk, when mixed with sesame seed milk, makes it approximate more the low protein content of mother's milk. Such a vegetable milk is much better, more alkaline and more digestible than almond milk or soybean milk, with their excessive protein content.

To make sesame seed milk, add hulled sesame seeds and water to a liquefier, adding less or more water to make a cream or a milk. The cream may be used as the base of a salad dressing or mayonnaise-substitute, valuable for those on alkaline diets who wish to avoid the acid-forming effects of vegetable oils and who yet desire some dressing over their salads. (It has been claimed that when salads are dressed with salad oils, especially refined oils, the acid-forming effect of the oil neutralizes the alkaline effect of the vegetables, so that the final reaction of the meal is an acid, rather than an alkaline, one. On the other hand, when sesame seed cream dressings, thus prepared, are used on salads, there is no acid effect.)

Sesame seed cream made in the manner above described by simply liquefying (using less water than to make sesame seed milk), may be used as the base of a cholesterol-free healthful ice cream, by simply mixing fruit pulp in it and then freezing in a refrigerator. (A similar sesame coconut or coconut cream may be made in the same way from sesame-coconut or coconut cream. Bananas, pistachio nuts, etc. may be added for extra flavor and nutritional value. Ice creams, thus prepared, are both delicious and nutritious.)

To make from sesame seeds a butter that resembles cow's butter, all that is necessary is to mix sesame seed cream with coconut oil (the natural, unrefined coconut oil which solidifies under low temperature) and place in a refrigerator. The sesame seed cream will add to the coconut the yellow color it lacks, or some carrot juice may be added to supply yellow carotene. (There is a product on the market, to which we already referred, "Soya Lecithin Butter", which is made from sesame seed, olive and soybean oils, with soya lecithin and carotene from carrots.)

Since sesame seeds are very rich in proteins and fats, it is best to use them in the form of dressings over other foods, as vegetables, cereals, etc., rather than to eat them by themselves. However, many people chew the hulled seeds. By placing them on a baking pan in an oven, at low temperature, until they dehydrate and become crisp, they are much easier to chew and digest, and are much tastier. They may then be easily crushed under a rolling pin into a meal, which is very delicious and digestible, providing a a non-acid-forming source of high quality proteins and fats in the diet. This sesame seed meal may be sprinkled over salads, cereals, vegetables, etc., as well as used in cooking and baking. The fresher it is made, the better the flavor and vitamin value, which becomes dissipated through oxidation on contact with air. For this reason, if stored, it should be kept in a closed airtight container, such as a glass jar with a tight cover which screws on. (It has been found that cornmeal, which otherwise becomes insect-infested in a relatively short time, if packed into a glass jar, which is closed airtight, may be kept as long as three years without spoiling.)

Hulled sesame seeds may be reduced to a meal with the aid of a liquefier, but the writer prefers the hand-rolling method, since less heat is generated and there is greater conservation of flavor and vitamins.

Sesame Seed Milk Versus Cow's Milk

Excellent substitutes for dairy products may be made from hulled sesame seeds by the aid of a good liquefier. They have the many advantages over cow's products which we have mentioned, namely, they are free from cholesterol, free from disease germs, free from putrefactive bacteria and tendency to constipate, free from mucus-forming properties, and rich in calciu, iron, phosphorus, high quality proteins, lecithin and vitamins. Either sesame seed milk or sesame-coconut milk are better both than cow's milk and than soybean milk, with its excessive protein content, resembling mother's milk more by their lower protein content. Like cow's milk, both sesame seed milk and coconut-sesame seed milk, turns in a clabber when it sours (and may even be made into a yogurt by addition of yogurt culture, though the writer sees no value in this, since the Bulgarian bacillus which forms yogurt does not find its native habitat in the human intestine, as does the acidophilic bacteria present in sour milk.

Many persons, both adults and infants, are allergic to cow's milk and cannot take its, without becoming bilious, constipated, have a white tongue, begin to expell mucus and suffer from various symptoms of the autointoxication which milk produces. The fact that cow's milk contains three times as much protein as mother's milk is one reason why it tends to constipate infants so readily, since this excessive protein tends to putrefy in the intestines, forming toxic putrefactive end-products which paralyze the intestinal muscles. While soybean milk is supposed to be anti-putrefactive, its very excessive protein content makes it undesirable as a substitute for mother's milk, whose protein content is very much less. How the infant, whose kidneys and organs were constructed for a fluid nutriment low in protein (mother's milk) can handle such a rich protein substance as soybean milk, the writer cannot understand. On the other hand, coconut milk has been very successfully employed for infant feeding throughout the tropics, its composition bearing greater resemblence to mother's milk, since it is low in protein, alkaline in reaction and rich in calcium, phosphorus and vitamins, as well as in vitamin D. which cow's milk lacks, especially in winter time, and which is essential for the health and normal growth of the infant. For all these reasons, coconut milk, or coconut-sesame seed milk, are superior to cow's milk, both for infants and adults.

Virgin Sesame Seed Oil and Tahini

"Tahini" is the name of an imported sesame seed cream dressing, coming from Turkey. It is the entire hulled seed crushed into a thick cream, which is used as a dressing over salads, vegetables, cereals, legumes, etc. It is a balanced and digestible fat, containing virgin sesame seed oil in combination with minerals, protein, etc.

A "Top-Tahini" cold pressed virgin sesame seed oil is now on the market, which is one of the most superior, digestible and delicious vegetable oils available. It is the natural sesame oil that rises to the of "Tahini" as it settles, and contains its full vitamin, lecithin and unsaturated fatty acid content. It is quite different from the usual types of sesame seed oil on the market, whether virgin or refined.

Throughout Turkey, Syria and other countries of the Near East, virgin sesame seed oil is a basic source of fat in the diet, in place of cholesterol-containing animal fats, which are known to cause hardening of the arteries, gall stones and cancer. In China, too, sesame seed oil, peanut oil and soybean oil are used in place of animal fats for all dietary purposes. It is a fact that cholesterol-caused diseases, including cancer, are comparatively rare among these races; which also possess unusual longevity and agility during advanced years. An example in afforded by Zaro, the Turk who was active and lively when a century and a half in age. His diet, as far as can be ascertained, was very low in cholesterol, consisting largely of sesame seed products, vegetables and fruits. It should be born in mind that in addition to being free from cholesterol, sesame seed products are rich in lecithin, which prevents the deposit of cholesterol by keeping it in solution.

Sunflower Seeds, The Miracle Food

The sunflower seed is Nature's treasure house of nutrition, being extremely rich in proteins, vitamins and minerals. Its protein content surpasses that of practically every other food known, being about three times as rich as meat and about 50% richer than the soybean. As a source of vitamin, weight for weight, than wheat germ. It also is a good source of vitamins A, D, E, and F. Its relatively high content of vitamin D is understandable when we consider that the sunflower turns to face the sun from its rising to its setting and so receives a maximum of ultra-violet rays, more so than the flowers of any other seeds, which lack this mobile capacity.

As a source of minerals, sunflower seeds are unique. It is known to farmers that the sunflower plant is a voracious mineral feeder and quickly depletes the mineral content of the soil in which it grows. Since Nature takes special provision to store a maximum supply of vitamins and minerals in seeds, for the support of the unborn seedling, we can understand why sunflower seeds are so rich in minerals, which include rare trace minerals that the deep roots of the sunflower plant brings up from deep in the soil. Among these trace minerals are magnesium, silicon and fluorine, all important for the formation of strong tooth enamel. It has been observed that Russians who are inveterate sunflower seed eaters, often nibbling on them all day long, tend to have large, strong bones and healthy, caries-free teeth, for sunflower seeds are rich in calcium and phosphorus, as well as in magnesium, silicon and fluorine, all of which minerals work together to form strong, hard teeth.

Sunflower seeds have played an important part in the diet of millions of Europeans and Orientals since time immemorial, supplying them with essential vitamins and minerals to help keep them in health and vigor. It may be observed that sunflower-seed eating races, as the Chinese and Russians are very prolific and fertile, showing no tendency to sterility due to lack of vitamin E.

The protein content of the sunflower seed varies from 31%, according to some figures, to 55%, according to others, though the latter is the one most generally accepted. Studies at the Agricultural Experiment Station of the University of Illinois have shown that sunflower seed kernel protein is 94% digestible and has high biological value.

Sunflower seeds are very rich in niacin, thiamin and other factors of the B complex. Sunflower seed kernel meal was found to contain five times as much thiamin as peanut meal and over six times as much as whole wheat. It contains about twice as much niacin as peanut meal and over five times as much as whole wheat. Not only are sunflower seeds richer in vitamin B complex than wheat germ, but are a better and safer source, because wheat germ, unless freshly milled tends to undergo rancid decomposition of its oil content, making it harder to digest and irritating to the gastro-intestinal tract. Sunflower seeds, being a whole, unmilled product, are free from this objection. They are also a better source of vitamin E than wheat germ oil, which, being highly concentrated, may be harmful if taken in excess and not under a physician's direction. Sunflower seeds, on the other hand, provide vitamin E in a safe form, without danger of excess.

The only danger in using an excess of sunflower seeds is to obtain too much protein, in which substance they are extremely rich. In this respect sesame seeds are superior, and to be preferred by those on low protein diets.

Other vitamins found in sunflower seeds are carotene, or pro-vitamin A, necessary for good eyesight, vitamin F (unsaturated fatty acids) and vitamin K, to which its anti-hemorrhagic property, noted by Rodale, the first to popularize sunflower seed eating in America about ten years ago, has observed in several instances (causing gum bleeding of pyorrhea to cease).

Sunflower seeds are valuable as a dietary source of fluorine; and those who are worried that the American people are not getting sufficient fluorine in their diet for teeth enamel will do well to add sunflower seeds and products to their diet rather than advaocate the mass poisoning of fluoridation, or the addition of inorganic sodium fluoride (a rat poison) to the water supplies of American cities. Much better than inorganic sodium fluoride is the <u>organic</u> fluorine of the sunflower seed.

Vitamin D is lacking in most vegetalbe foods, so it is comforting to the vegetarian to know that he may obtain this vitamin from sunflower seeds and does not have to use fish liver oil to obtain it in winter time.

Sunflower seeds may be eaten from the shell, but they are tastiest when slightly toasted over a pan or in the oven, which makes them crisp and crunchy and easier to remove from the shell. They are also available in shelled form; and in this case too, they are best when first placed on a baking pan in an oven under low temperature until they become crisp and crunchy, in which form they are easier to chew and digest than when raw, for the raw seeds have a rubbery consistency. After being dehydrated in this manner the kernels are easier to crush under a rolling pin into a meal, though the raw kernel may also be crushed without difficulty. Sunflower seed meal may be sprinkled over foods to enrich them with organic minerals and natural vitamins, as well as high quality proteins.

Vegetable Meat Substitute Made from Sunflower Seeds

From sunflower seed meal, a wonderful meat substitute may be made, which looks and tastes like meat. To prepare this, first cook lentils (preferably organic Turkish red split or green lentils, or South American lentils) and then mash them, adding sunflower seed meal (also sesame seed meal if desired). Add sage, majoram, basil or other culinary herbs, and some grated onions, garlic, ground celery seeds and other ingredients of a vegetable meat loaf. The mixture may be baked as a loaf, then sliced, and served with a tomato sauce, or made into patties and placed over a griddle. The reddish color of the lentils and the brown color of sunflower seed meal give a meat-like appearance, while the heating of sunflower and sesame seed meals gives off an odor that is remarkably meat-like. Those who wish a protein substitute for meat will be delighted with this sunflower seed meat substitute. (This recipe can of course be varied and undoubtedly improved.)

The writer first learned of the capacity of sunflower seeds, in the form of a meal, to provide the base for a vegetable meat substitute from a California dietitian, who prepared a sunflower meat loaf (which was first baked and then sliced and prepared as patties and served with a tomato sauce) that looked, tasted and even smelled so much like meat that it even deceived maggots, for once when it was placed outside to cool, maggots promptly collected around it, as they do around meat.

One marked advantage of this sunflower meat substitute (which can prepared together with sesame seed and pepitoria squash seed meal, plus of course mashed cooked lentils and other ingredients), over meat itself, besides its lower cost, is the fact that while it supplies nearly three times as much complete protein of high biological value and all essential amino acids otherwise found in meat (especially when sunflower seeds are supplemented by sesame and pepitoria squash seeds), it is bacteria-free, and does not contain disease germs or putrefactife bacteria, not to mention uric acid and toxic extractives, usually found in meat. For this reason it does not tend to produce intestinal putrefaction or cause constipation as meat does. It is a far more healthful food. Also it is most delicious and highly nutritious, for while meat supplies little more than protein (except uric acid, urea, creatin and toxic extractives that give it is characteristic taste and which are really stimulants, rather than supplying any real nutrition), and is highly acid-forming, this meat substitute is rich in alkaline minerals and vitamins, including calcium, magnesium, iron, etc.

Virgin sunflower seed oil has been a basic source of fat in the diet of the Russian peasantry for centuries; and is now available in this country for the first time. It is quite different from tasteless refined sunflower seed oil, since it has a deep golden color and a characteristic sunflower seed flavor and aroma. It is considered more digestible and superior to the finest virgin olive oil, being less acid-forming. (Olive oil, in spite of being so highly praised, has the highest acidity and is consequently one of the least digestible, of all vegetable oils. Whether this is due to the fact that the olive, from which it is desired, contains considerable tannic acid, or due to some other source of acidity, the writer is not certain. In any event, sesame seed and sunflower seed oils are much less acid and are more digestible.)

Pepitoria Squash Seeds:
Ancient Food of the Maya Indians

These are a basic food of the Maya Indians of Guatemala, who have used them for centuries. These seeds come from a special squash, grown only for its seeds, and whose flesh is not edible. Indians shell them by hand, and the kernels are sold in most Indian markets. These kernels are toasted, stone-ground into a meal and then added to foods. The toasted kernel is sold in Mexico as a delicacy, like we sell roasted peanuts.

The Maya Indians seem to prefer pepitoria squash seeds to sesame seeds, and sesame seeds to sunflower seeds, which they do not grow at all. Both pepitoria squash seeds and sesame seeds are used in their diet, in the manner described above. The writer has added pepitoria squash seeds to his diet while traveling through Central America, and was delighted. In fact, after he started to use them, he could not think of using sesame sunflower seeds - they were so superior in so many ways. First of all they are lower in protein, and hence more digestible than sunflower seeds, since all proteins involve considerable expenditure of digestive energy. Also they seemed to have a more alkaline effect; and when "popped" by toasting, were extremely crunchy and delicious. While Indians crush the kernels into a meal by stone, one can do the same with a rolling pin. The meal is excellent added to soups, giving them a spicy flavor.

There is on the market squash seeds imported from Turkey, and also pumpkin seeds. These are best toasted, in which form they are eaten from the shell as a delicacy. One advantage of eating sunflower seeds, squash seeds and pumpkin seeds from the shell is that their full vitamin content and flavor is retained, more so than in the case of the shelled seed, whose kernel has been exposed to the air. Another advantage is that there is then less tendency to overeat, due to the time and labor involved in removing the seeds from the shell, since seeds are very concentrated foods and should be eaten in moderation. In general, the writer finds squash and pumpkin seeds to be the best of all seeds. They are larger, easier to chew and digest, and lower in protein. (The writer advocates a low protein diet as best for physical and mental efficiency.

Hemp Seeds

It has been reported that the people of India prefer hemp seeds to sesame seeds, because of their pronounced flavor, which is somewhat aromatic. In Turkey they are preferred because of their high value as a re-constituent, and are used by persons who are run down and need building up. They are extremely rich in vitamins. The seeds have a hard shell and when eaten whole are less tasty than other seeds, for which reason they should be stone-crushed into a meal. (When machine-ground, sharp parts of the hull remain in the meal, which should be strained to remove them.) Undoubtedly hemp seeds are best in the form of an oil. Due to the fact that marijuana is extracted from hemp seed, just as opium is obtained from poppy seed, all hemp seeds sold in this country must be sterilized by law, so that they may not be used for planting purposes. However, the writer has found nothing objectionable about the use of hemp seeds, and noticed no harmful effects. On the other hand, they seemed to be exceptionally rich in vitamins.

Canteloupe Seeds
For Making Vegetable Milk and Dairy Products

Of all seeds, canteloupe seeds make a vegetable milk and dairy product substitutes that most resemble cow's milk and its products. One reason for this is because of their low protein content relatively higher calcium content (in relation to protein). (Sunflower seeds, with their excessive protein content, for this reason, is not adapted for milk making, though it makes one of the best meat substitutes.) By means of a liquefier, canteloupe seeds (either the moist fresh seeds or dried seeds that have been soaked) can be made into an excellent milk which, when it sours, greatly resembles sour cow's milk, forming a similar clabber, from which a cholesterol-free, bacteria-free, non-putrefactive cottage cheese may be made. It may be noted in passing that though cottage cheese has been highly praised as a source of calcium, since most cottage cheese on the market were made from pasteurized milk and since the pasteurization process renders most of its calcium unavailable for physiological use, cottage cheese is not a good source of calcium, and neither are the salted older cheeses, since salt has a decalcifying effect, with the result that though chemical analysis may show such cheeses to be rich in calcium, their effect on the body is not only to add no calcium, but even to withdraw body calcium.

During his travels through Central America, the writer noticed that the Indians appreciated the value of melon seeds and carefully saved them when they opened melons, and made a milk and cream from them which they added to their foods. They crushed the seeds by stone crushers, mixed them with water and then strained out the refuse. In Turkey, Syria and other countries of the Near East melon seeds are similarly employed, and are even imported to this country for use by the Turkish and Syrian population here. In general, Orientals are far more advanced in appreciation and knowledge of the nutritional value of seeds than Occidentals; and it is probably by their use of seeds that they have been able so successfully to be vegetarians, often strict vegetarians (using no dairy products), as are the Chinese. Prof. McCollum of Johns Hopkins University has stated that his experiments have shown that for a vegetarian diet to be successful, seeds should be incorporated in the diet, and that for one to obtain sufficient calcium without using dairy products it is necessary to use plenty of greens.

Flaxseed tea has long been used as a medicine, for constipation, having a lubricating action on the intestines. Flaxseed meal makes an excellent poultice in cases of inflammation, boils, etc. An infusion is useful in catarrhal conditions of the bronchial tubes and also of the urinary organs. It has a soothing and strengthening action on the kidneys and bladder. Among the Indians of the Andes, stone-crushed flaxseed meal (with some toasted barley mixed with the meal to present it from becoming too fatty) is used, as well as sesame seed meal, similarly prepared. The writer had occasion to eat these seed meals while traveling through the Andes and found them highly nutritious as well as delicious. They are best freshly made, deteriorating rapidly as all vital substances do.

Flaxseed meal is rich in vitamin F (linoleic acids of the linseed oil it contains), and therefore may be used for cooking and baking in place of other fats and refined shortenings. Flaxseed meal is excellent added to baked products, giving them laxative properties, and this is also true of foods cooked with it.

From flaxseed a highly nutritious oil is made, known as linseed oil, which is widely used in Germany as a cooking and salad oil, being rich in lecithin and vitamins, especially vitamin F. Though in this country it is used for paint manufacture, this does not mean it is not a highly nutritious and healthful oil, as is the case with soybean oil, which is also used for manufacture of automobile paint.

Anise Seed

This seed has long been used both for culinary and medicinal uses. It is used as a flavoring agent in baking cakes. A decoction of anise seeds has long been used to relieve pains and colic in small children. Anise has a quieting and soothing effect on the stomach, stimulating its action. It is believed to increase milk secretion in nursing mothers, as dill seed also is. (Ground dill seed is used to flavor food; it is rich in vitamins and adds value to foods which it seasons.)

Fennel Seeds

Tea of these seeds is used for colds and coughs and for wind colic in children, also for spasms.

Mahlep Seed

This seed imported from Turkey, when ground and added to baked products, gives them a most delicious cake-like flavor, and is in great demand by bakers aware of its flavoring properties.

Coriander Seed

This seed, ground, makes a healthful, delightful natural seasoning agent for many foods, though generally used for cakes.

Cumin Seed

This seed is widely used in the Near East for seasoning foods.

Achiote Seed

This red, tropical seed is used to impart a yellow color to foods with which it is cooked. It is popular in Central and South America, and is mostly used to color rice, though it is also used to color other foods as well. Studies have shown that it is very rich in vitamins and is worthy of more careful study as a possible source of nutritional essentials that may be lacking in most diets. In Guatemala, some time ago, a firm was established which was devoted to the production and exportation of ground achiote seed as a dietary vitamin supplement.

Watermelon Seeds

From watermelon seeds was extracted a substance that has proven very valuable in the treatment of kidney diseases. It aids the kidneys to perform their function more effectively.

CHAPTER EIGHT

ORGANIC FOODS FOR BETTER HEALTH

As time goes on, more and more health-conscious people are demanding Organic Foods, and realizing that their health can be safeguarded in no other way. Dr. W. Coda Martin writes: "Organic foods have 20 to 40 per cent greater vitamin and trace mineral content than those grown in depleted soils." (He should add, "by the use of chemical fertilizers and sprays, which further deteriorate their health-giving value, and may indeed make them disease-producing.") We shall now describe the nutritional value of several outstanding Organic Foods. (These are distributed by Organic Food Research Associates, 215 Sixth Street, Lorian, Ohio.)

ORGANICALLY GROWN FIGS AS ANTI-ANEMIC FOODS

It is not generally known that figs are unique in the vegetable kingdom because of their extraordinary content of blood-building constituents - including high quantities of two anti-anemic vitamins - vitamin B-12 and folic acid - as well as iron and copper, which are so important for hemoglobin regeneration. It is fortunate that organically grown figs are now available, from two sources: California and Turkey. For the vegetarian who may worry that he may not secure enough iron for his blood if he gives up meat, it should be remembered that the iron of meat which exists in association with a high content of copper and the two anti-anemic vitamins just mentioned, while inorganic iron compounds have been found to be worthless and even harmful, since the body cannot use iron in inorganic form. Hence, the folly to "enrich" bread and flours with inorganic iron. Only plants can use inorganic iron as exists in the soil. Animals and humans must obtain their iron in organic combination as prepared by plants and cannot assimilate iron directly from nature in its inorganic form. Otherwise we should swallow iron filings, or, if they are too irritating, scrape off some iron rust from an old water pipe, dissolve it in water and drink it, if we have anemia. We all know that such inorganic iron will be more or less poisonous and that the body cannot use it.

The ancient Romans held figs in high esteem. This Pliny (70 A.D.) wrote: "Figs are restorative and the best food for those who are brought low by sickness, and are on their way to recover. They increase the strength of young people, and preserve the elderly in better health and make them look younger and with fewer wrinkles. They are so nutritive as to cause corpulency and strength; for this cause professional wrestlers and champions were in times past fed with figs."

Recent researches on the nutritional value of figs have confirmed Pliny's view. They have shown that figs are exceptionally rich in vitamins and minerals necessary for the formation and regeneration of red blood cells, perhaps richer than any other member of the fruit kingdom, with the possible exception of the pomegranate, whose reputation as a blood purifier and builder depended on more than the fact that its deep red juice resembles blood.

FIGS AS SOURCES OF VITAMIN B-12, FOLIC ACID, COPPER, IRON, ETC.

The studies of Dr. Agnes Fay Morgan at the University of California have shown that dried figs contain .032 mg. per cent vitamin B-12, the so-called "animal protein factor", which is good news for vegetarians, who might think that they might suffer a lack of this vitamin, which most vegetable foods do not contain, in such large amounts. In addition to this anti-anemic vitamin, Dr. Morgan found figs rich in another anti-anemic vitamin, also a member of the B complex, folic acid. And what is more remarkable, she found them also rich in blood-building minerals that act in conjunction with these vitamins in hemoglobin formation: copper (3.5% mg.) and iron (.0031%), more than is contained in spinach. This complex of minerals and vitamins makes figs very valuable for anemia. Recently a new product has been put in the market known as "Figpep", which is the concentrated juice of figs, prepared by a special process which preserves the vitamins and minerals of figs, and creates a stable product, without the use of preservatives. "Figpep" is a natural alkalizer. (It is distributed by Organic Food Research Associates, 215 Sixth Street, Lorain, Ohio.) Addition of water converts this fig syrup into a tasty beverage, which laxative qualities, due to the presence of a laxative substance, diaphenzyl isatin, which is naturally present in figs (also prunes, which contain about half the quantity). Since figs and this concentrated fig syrup are alkaline in reaction, while prunes, like plums and cranberries are acid-forming (due to the presence of benzoic acid, which reduces to hippuric acid in the body, in which form it is given off through the urine), they are to be preferred as natural fruit laxatives. Black mission figs are excellent when soaked overnight and the dark juice used as a morning beverage. It is tasty, nutritious and laxative. (Be sure to use organically grown, unsulphured figs and glass-distilled water.)

Dried figs are good sources of five B vitamins. They are an unusually good source of thiamin and folic acid. They also contain riboflavin, niacin and pantothetic acid in appreciable amounts, as well as folic acid and B-12, as has previously been mentioned.

Figs are an excellent source of calcium and phosphorus. They contain twice as much calcium as cow's milk, are rich in alkaline minerals which help counteract acidosis, and contain a proteolytic enzyme known as ficin, which helps in digesting proteins. They have a small amount of carotene and vitamin C.

Dr. Morgan, in experimental tests on children, conducted at Berkeley, California, found that four figs per day showed up almost twice the benefit of milk used in a supplemental diet and far better than oranges and other items tried.

IMPORTED ALKALINE NUTS
Pine Nuts, Chestnuts, Pistachio Nuts, Filberts and Coconuts
Acid-Forming Nuts: Peanuts, Walnuts, Pecans

We may divide nuts into two groups: Domestic Acid-forming Nuts, which are less desirable, and the Imported Alkaline Nuts, which are more desirable, and the best to use.

Domestic Acid-Forming Nuts include walnuts, pecans and peanuts. These are grown with chemical fertilizers, and they may be sprayed. After harvesting they are fumigated. California walnuts and almonds are bleached. Fumigation poisons have been shown to penetrate through the thin shell of the almond and be found in the kernel.

Peanuts are the most acid-forming of all nuts. They contain uric acid and they form additional uric acid in the system through the metabolic breakdown of their protein. Peanut butter, therefore, is acid-forming. Sesame seed butter is far superior, being richer in minerals, and though richer in protein, is alkaline in reaction.

Walnuts are very acid-forming. Their skin contains tannic acid, as does the skin of pecans, almonds, pistachios and filberts. But when the skins of almonds, pistachios and filberts can be removed by blanching, that of the walnut and filbert, due to the conboluted shape of the kernel, cannot easily be removed. The characteristically bitter taste of walnuts and pecans is due to the large amount of tannic acid they contain. (Tannic acid is a toxic substance found in tea; it is astringent and constipating.) Pecans are a little better than walnuts, but have the same objections.

Imported Alkaline Nuts include Italian pine nuts and chestnuts, Spanish almonds, Turkish filberts, pistachios, which come from various countries of the Near East, and tropical coconuts. These nuts are all better than the acid-forming ones mentioned. They should be used in their place. Coming from distant lands where agriculture is more natural and primitive and where chemical fertilizers and sprays are not so apt to be employed, they are safer to use. The pine nut, in particular, is not likely to be either fertilized or sprayed, since the pine tree is a hardy tree which is not attacked by insects. The same applies to the coconut, which is fertilized by marine trace minerals, carried to it by wind-borne sea spray, rainfall and subterranean. (See page from the ocean) since it will not produce away from the sea. The coconut is one of the safest foods sold in American markets, and though the writer heard of a practice of removing coconut water and replacing it with ordinary water to prevent spoilage of coconuts, and also heard of chemical fertilizers being employed on commercial coconut crops in the Phillipines, in general it is less likely to be contaminated with chemicals than other nuts or foods.

While peanuts, cashews and pine nuts are called "nuts", they are really not nuts at all. The peanut is an underground legume, possessing the uric-acid-forming tendency of several other legumes, but to a higher extent, because lower in alkaline minerals and more acid-forming. The pine nut is really the seed of the pine tree, growing in clusters in pine cones, as seeds grow, rather than individually, as true nuts and fruits do. The cashew is the seed of the cashew fruit, which grows external to, and adjacent to the fruit. In its raw form it is highly poisonous and is avoided by tropical natives, unless roasted in the shell over a flame, whereupon its highly inflammable and poisonous oil burns, and so it is de-poisoned to a large extent. But when the raw cashew is shelled and shipped to this country, it is impossible to get rid of its poison, achieved only by the burning of the oil present between the kernel and the shell in which it is encased. It is therefore best to avoid cashews, though if eaten they should be thoroughly toasted, as heat tends to drive out the poison, though it is doubtful if this can be done after the raw kernel is removed from the shell.

Almonds are generally rated as the most alkaline nut, when, as a matter of fact, they are the least alkaline member of the alkaline group, due to their high content of acid-forming protein elements in proportion to their small amount of alkaline minerals. On the other hand, in the chestnut the protein content is much lower and the alkaline mineral content much higher; and the same is true of the filbert, pistachio, pine nut and coconut, all of which are more alkaline and better than the almond, especially when the almond is not blanched and thus freed from its tannic-acid-containing shell. (Much of the digestive difficulty that people find after eating nuts is due to the intake of tannic acid present in the skin of nuts, which should never be eaten. The pine nut is free from tannic acid because its skin does not adhere to the kernel but comes off after the nut is shelled, pine nuts being usually sold in skinless shelled form. For this reason, but its more highly alkaline reaction in general, the pine nut should be preferred to the almond, even when blanched. It is softer to properly chew and more digestible.

The filbert is lower in protein and more alkaline and digestible than the almond. Like other nuts with skins, it should be first blanched and then placed in an oven under low temperature until it becomes thoroughly dry and crisp Seeds and nuts, so eaten, are much more digestible than in their moist raw form, which gives them a somewhat rubbery consistency, making them harder to chew. In this respect the more delicious taste of the dry, crisp, slightly toasted seed and nut (not roasted or heated sufficiently to destroy vitamins), is a good juice.

Nuts being very rich in protein and fat, are somewhat one-sided foods and should not be eaten freely or alone. The only nut that can safely be eaten alone and which can provide the base for a satisfactory mono diet is the chestnut, because it is so well balanced by having much smaller amounts of protein and fat and much more carohydrates than other nuts, which lack sufficient carbohydrates to balance their excessive protein and fat content. For that reason they are best eaten with dried fruits, as dates, figs and raisins, which supply carbohydrates to balance their protein and fats. Otherwise nuts, like pine nuts and coconuts, should be made into a cream and used as a dressing over other foods, as salads, cereals, etc. So used there is less tendency to overeat on them than when eaten alone.

NUTRITIONAL VALUE OF PINE NUTS

Pine nuts are one of the most alkaline, digestible and finest of all nuts. Their soft consistency makes them easier to chew up into a cream and to properly assimilate. They are light on the digestive organs because they do not tend to be swallowed in small pieces, as some of the other harder nuts when they are not properly masticated, but also because they are free from any tannic-acid-containing skin, as the almond has, and which makes nuts more acid than they otherwise would be (for which reason blanched nuts are more alkaline, the pine nut being naturally blanched and not requiring any heating treatment as applied for the blanching of other nuts). Recognition of the high alkaline reaction and nutritive value of the pine nut has made it the preferred nut for diabetics, diabetes being a disease of acid intoxication for which acid-forming nuts would be objectionable.

Pine nuts provide one of the finest proteins in the diet, supplying an amino acid equivalent of meat, eggs and milk. It is claimed by biologists that in prehistoric times, the pine nut was the first and original nut to be consumed by mammals, since pine trees flourished at that time. Even so-called carnivorous animals are believed to have once depended on pine nuts for their protein before a geological cataclysm deprived them of their natural food and forced them to change their habitat and diet.

Those who have difficulty in digesting other nuts, especially those with tannic-acid-containing skins will find pine nuts perfectly agreeable, since they are entirely free from tannic acid.

There are two chief varieties of pine nuts used for food in this country, the pignolia nut imported from Italy, and the pinon pine, known as the Indian nut (because picked by Indians in the Southwest where it grows wild). However the latter crop is sporadic and often is not available, whereas the pignolia nut may be had most of the time, and hence is the one most commonly sold. Since the pine tree is a hardy tree, requiring no chemical fertilization or spraying, the pine nut fulfills all organic requirements and is worthy to be classed among Organic Super Foods.

Pine nuts may be eaten as they are, together with organically grown figs, raisins or dates; and they are extra crunchy and delicious when first thoroughly dried in an oven at a sufficiently low temperature so as not to destroy their vitamins. In either form, they are easily crushed under a rolling pin into a meal, which may be sprinkled over salads, vegetables, cereals, etc., or mixed with soups, supplying one of the most digestible and alkaline sources of protein and fat in the diet, as well as considerable organic calcium, magnesium and iron.

Another way to prepare pine nuts is to make them into a milk or cream by the aid of a liquefier. Such a pine nut cream makes a delicious, alkaline, digestible salad dressing for use by those who wish to avoid use of acid-forming vegetable oils, which, as we have already pointed out, may turn an otherwise alkaline salad to have a final acid reaction on the body. In general, nuts, like seeds, being very rich in proteins and fats, and consequently one-sided, should not be eaten freely, and especially not eaten alone, but used in limited amounts combined with dried fruits, as dressings over salads, cereals, etc.

Chestnuts, the Most Alkaline and Balanced of All Nuts

As we have already pointed out, the chestnut is the only nut so well balanced in its composition, as well as alkaline in reaction, that it can serve as a balanced meal in itself, while in the case of other nuts, even if considered alkaline, they have an excess of acid-forming proteins and fats and insufficient carbohydrates and alkaline minerals to balance them. While they require carbohydrates, as dates, figs or raisins, to balance them, the chestnut contains its own carbohydrates and needs no balancing. Roasted chestnuts make a nutritious and satisfying meal with an alkaline reaction. An exclusive chestnut diet makes an excellent mono diet.

The chestnut is unique among nuts in being a carbohydrate food, or at least may be used as such. In Italy, where the chestnuts are an important crop (chestnuts sold in this country being largely imported from Italy, since blight has destroyed most of the American crop), they are ground into a flour which is used in baking. Chestnut flour being alkaline in reaction should be more widely used in baking, especially for persons who are allergic to acid-forming flours, as wheat. Millet flour is another alkaline flour which should be more widely used to counteract the acid effects of wheat and rye flour. A professor in a college in the central part of the United States, after learning how millet saved the lives of millions during the famine that followed the first world war, became interested in millet, which he prepared as a flour and gave to several women he knew to try in baking. He found that addition of millet flour to baked products greatly improved the flavor, alkalinity and vitamin and mineral content of bread and cookies; also millet, containing a complete protein, balanced the incomplete profits of other grains. Both chestnut flour and millet flour should be more widely used to replace and balance acid-forming wheat and rye flours.

Chestnuts are best roasted, though they are sometimes used cooked or steamed. While the fresh chestnut, unlike other nuts, are perishable and cannot be stored when out of season, dried shelled chestnuts are available the year round. They should be soaked in water and then cooked as an alkaline carbohydrates to replace acid-forming grains. They may also be used in place of sprayed potatoes.

Pistachio Nuts, the Only Nut With a Green Flesh

The pistachio nut is the only green-fleshed nut, the green color of the kernel suggesting a high mineral content and alkalinity. Just what substance it contains, whether chlorophyl or something else, that makes it green, to the writer's knowledge, has never been determined. At any rate, the pistachio is one of the superior alkaline nuts. While practically all pistachios in the shell have been soaked in brine and contain salt adhering to their kernel, it is possible now to secure unsalted, uncolored pistachios. They are best when toasted, whereupon the tannic-acid-containing red skin covering the green kernel easily peels off when the nut is shelled.

Turkish Filberts

Filberts are one of the superior alkaline nuts, which are better than the acid-forming nuts described above, and better than almonds, which are much richer in protein and therefore less alkaline and digestible. Imported Turkish filberts are more likely to be raised in a natural manner than American-grown nuts. Filberts are best when blanched dried in an oven until crisp.

Coconuts, King of Nuts

Researches by Cajori and others have shown that nuts contain complete proteins which can replace animal proteins, including meat, eggs and milk. Of all nuts tested, the coconut was found to contain a protein of the highest biological value, surpassing not only that of other nuts but also meat, eggs and milk.

Young growing animals were found to undergo a <u>supernormal</u> rate of growth when fed on coconut protein, greater than that produced by milk protein. A South American scientist announced that coconut milk provides a perfect substitute for mother's milk; and throughout the tropics infants which cannot nurse are successfully raised on coconut milk in place of mother's milk. Its low protein content, high alkalinity and richness in minerals and vitamins makes it an ideal nutriment for young growing organisms after weaning.

How to Make Coconut Milk, Cream, Oil, and Butter

The coconut is undoubtedly one of the best nuts, provided properly prepared and used. Few people know that the meat of the coconut should really be eaten when in the soft jelly stage, before it hardens, when it is much less digestible. Those unable to properly chew and digest the solid flesh of the ripe coconut should grate it and then squeeze the grated coconut through a cheesecloth. From each coconut, a cup of coconut cream can be thus squeezed out. By dipping in some warm water or keeping in hot steam, it becomes easier to squeeze the maximum amount of cream from the grated coconut. Mixing the cream with coconut water, one secures coconut milk. Thus from each coconut one can secure about two glasses of coconut milk.

Another way to make coconut cream and milk is by means of a liquefier. Simply add pieces of coconut or grated coconut to the liquefier, with water, varying the amount of water to make either coconut milk or coconut cream.

If fresh coconut is not available, shredded coconut or coconut meal may be liquefied to make coconut milk or cream. In this case be sure to obtain a dried coconut which was not treated with glycerine or other preservatives, as most such coconut products on the market have been.

Coconut cream makes an excellent alkaline salad dressing to replace acid-forming vegetable oils. It may also be used with cereals, in place of cholesterol-containing butter or cream. It may be added to baked products or used in cooking in place of other fats. Many tropical races cook in coconut milk, which gives foods a delicious fatty taste due to the release of coconut oil from the milk during cooking. The writer has known a young lady who was unalbe to stand the acid effects of vegetable oils and who did all her cooking with coconut milk and cream, as well as used coconut cream for a salad dressing. She claimed that she had no acid effects from it, whereas other fats, as vegetable oils, butter, etc., proved quite acid-forming.

To make a delicious home-made coconut ice cream, mix fruit pulp and banana with coconut cream and freeze in a refrigerator.

Coconut oil is uncoubtedly the most digestible and least acid-forming of all vegetable oils, especially when unrefined and made from the fresh coconut in the following manner. Reduce several coconuts to coconut cream or milk and add to about a quart of boiling water and boil until the oil rises to the top. The longer the water boils, the greater the amount of coconut oil on top in proportion to water below. The coconut oil may then be removed with a spoon, until completely removed.

This oil solidifies when the temperature drops and may then be used as a butter. It is one of the most digestible of all fats and may be used on salads, in cooking or baking or for the skin or hair. Foods fried in coconut oil are more digestible than when other more acid-forming oils are used.

Persons who suffer from acidosis will do well to use coconut cream, made from fresh coconut, in place of acid-forming vegetable oils, oleomargarine and butter.

The Coconut Water Regimen Versus Fasting

While the water of the coconut is often called "coconut milk", we here use the latter term to mean the cream derived from the meat of the coconut diluted with coconut water, or the fluid inside the coconut. This, however, is really not pure water, but contains in low concentration all the elements of the coconut meat, so that it is really a dilute coconut milk. An exclusive regimen of this coconut water, continued for long periods of time, has been found to have great therapeutic value. Throughout the tropics, where coconut water is taken daily as a beverage, its healthful properties are widely recognized, and it is especially used for the relief of kidney and bladder ailments, since it tends to fulsh and purify these organs and promote their healing. It also acts as general blood purifier, helping to neutralize acid toxins and remove impurities. A Jersey City physician achieved remarkable results with an exclusive coconut water regimen. In one case a woman with advanced consumption, given up to die, regained her health after living on coconut water alone for six months. In another case an infant, unable to take milk or any other nourishment, was fed on coconut water six months and thrived wonderfully, regaining its health. This is understandable, since coconut water provides a balanced form of nourishment, containing coconut proteins, fats, carbohydrates, minerals and vitamins, all in solution in the purest distilled water. Also it contains trace minerals which the coconut derives from the sea, and which most other foods lack. When liberal amounts of coconut water are taken, not only does one obtain the purifying and therapeutic of a fast, but at the same time one is kept well nourished, without having to experience the disagreealbe symptoms of a complete fast, involving extreme loss of weight and strength, but can continue one's normal life and activities. Also, while during a fast, lacking the food stimulus, perisitalsis stops and the intestinal contents stagmate, a coconut water regimen keeps the bowels free and open. And coconut water is purer than any other water that one may use during a fast. Should one use ordinary chemicalized city water, the harm it does can be greater than any benefits of a fast.

Sprouts For Vitamins

How to Sprout Mung Beans, Alfalfa Seeds, Sunflower Seeds, Chick Peas, Cress Seeds, Soy Beans, etc.

For centuries the Chinese peasants, in winter time, sprouted mung beans and used them in place of fresh vegetables, when these were not available. The Chinese practice of using bean sprouts was never given much attention by nutritionists until it was disdovered that the sprouting process develops vitamin C in legumes and seeds, even when this vitamin was absent from the unsprouted ones;

and whatever vitamins they contain are increased by sprouting. Some years ago, an American scientist, Brown Landone, developed an interest in the nutritional value of sprouted mung beans and performed experiments on rats. Two groups were fed on the same diet, except that sprouted mung beans were given to one group and not to the other. Landone claims that the rats that received the bean sprouts were reactivated, the older rats acquiring the characteristics of youth. It seemed that there was something present in these sprouts that had an energizing action on the endocrine glands, causing the rats to be rejuvenated.

Further studies revealed that sprouted seeds and legumes not only developed vitamins absent from unsprouted ones, but plant hormones known as auxins. These hormones seem to have a vitalizing action on cell life and activity. Gardeners apply them to cuttings to stimulate root development after transplanting. Landone believed that the auxins of sprouted mung beans, when eaten by animals or humans, stimulated cell activity, especially of the endocrine glands.

Believing that the auxins of sprouts, since they rejufenated rats, would preserve youth and prolong life in the case of man, Landone added them to his diet and used them daily. Though he was a heavy smoker and meat-eater, and paid no special attention to his diet, he lived to be nearly a hundred, and before his death looked like a man in his forties.

Landone's pioneer work on the value of sprouted foods was continued by others, who sprouted various other seeds, including alfalfa seeds, chick peas (garbanzos), soy beans, cress, etc. Alfalfa seeds make vitamin-rich sprouts which may be added to various foods and may be used in place of sprayed vegetables as a source of vitamins and minerals. (The victim of a "poisoned world", in which all available vegetables have been contaminated by sprays, would od well to remember that just as the Chinese peasants live all winter, and keep well, by using sprouted mung beans in place of fresh vegetables, they can very well follow their example and use sprouted seeds and legumes in place of poisoned fresh vegetables.

To sprout alfalfa seeds, sunflower seeds, mung beans, etc., first soak overnight and then spread on top of several layers of moistened cheesecloth, and covering with damp cheesecloth. Put in a warm dark place and keep continually damp by sprinkling water above. It will be well to place the layers of cheesecloth over a board with holes through the bottom or in a kitchen sink strainer or collander, so that the water added above may drain from the bottom.

A second method of sprouting is to place the soaked seeds in a flower pot, leaving enough room for them to expand as they sprout. Cover with a cheesecloth and add water from time to time to keep the seeds moist. If a flower pit is not available you may put the beans or seeds in a milk bottle or tall jar and tie some cheesecloth over the opening. Pour in water twice or more often each day and reverse the jar so that the water drains through the cheesecloth. In a few days you should have sprouts forming.

Sunflower seeds make excellent vitamin-rich sprouts, which may be sprinkled over salads. This is one of the finest ways to use sunflower seeds.

In the case of chick peas or garbanzos, which usually take a long time to cook, by first sprouting, the cooking time is greatly diminished. An excellent way to prepare sprouted legumes at all, but to add them to a pot of wild rice, millet, vegetables, etc. toward the end of cooking or after turning off the flame, letting them steam on top of the cooked food with lid on the pot, so that they tenderize in the steam. In this way their vitamins are retained to a greater extent than if they were cooked. Some prefer to eat all sprouts raw, adding the raw sprouts to cooked foods. This is undoubtedly best, for their life-giving elements are then retained to the fullest extent.

Cress seeds may be sprinkled over a dampened cheesecloth and left to sprout and grew into small tender cress leaves in a short time. Such young tender greens are much richer in vitamins than fully matured vegetables and infinitely more healthful than sprayed vegetables containing DDT, chlordane and other insecticide residues.

Organically minded city dweelers who wish to avoid use of chemically fertilized, sprayed vegetables and fruits will do well to establish a "kitchen sprout garden", growing various kinds of sprouts - alfalfa, mung bean, soy bean, chick pea, cress, sunflower seed, etc. and at different stages of development, so that fresh sprouts of different kinds will be available each day for incorporation in the diet, to supply vitamins in place of fresh vegetables. Studies on the vitamin content of sprouts have shown that the vitamins present in seeds originally (and seeds in general contain practically all vitamins) are increased in quantity by the process of sprouting.

In the case of the soy bean, when sprouted it is not only quicker to cook, but easier to digest; and the excessive protein content of the raw soy bean seems to be reduced in the sprouted one, for which reason persons who cannot handle unsprouted soy beans may find sprouted ones more agreeable.

In parts of the Tennessee, sprouted chick peas have been popular and were eaten raw, supplying valuable minerals and vitamins that might otherwise be lacking in the diet.

In India, yogis for since time immemorial recognized the value of sprouted foods and made it a practice to sprout millet and other grains before using, clamining that sprouted grains were much more healthful than unsprouted ones.

Persons who wish to avoid the use of chemically fertilized, sprayed vegetables and fruits will do well to use various sprouted seeds and legumes instead - including sprouted sunflower seeds, mung beans, chick peas, etc. In addition to sprouts, young tender greens of alfalfa and cress seedlings may be used. Here is a new interesting field for experimentation, to determine how many different seeds may be suitable as sources of vitamins, in sprouted form or in the fomr of young green leaves. The possibilities ar unlimited.

Dried corn makes excellent sprouts and so do other cereals.

Vitamin assays have shown that young tender greens of cereals, when a few days old, are higher in vitamins than the more mature plant or the grains. This is in accordance with the general rule that young organisms have more vitality than older ones. Therefore there is no reason why the person who wishes to avoid the use of sprayed green vegetables may not be able to secure his vitamins and minerals from sprouts and young tender alfalfa greens and other young tender greens instead.

How to Grow Parsley in Your Kitchen

Parsley has been found to be richer in vitamins and minerals than practically all other vegetables, especially in iron. In fact parsley has been found to contain high quantities of practically all important vitamins. While parsley as generally purchased on the market has little flavor and is often withered (besides not being perfectly safe, because even if not sprayed, it may be contaminated by DDT, chlordane, etc. by growing on land contaminated by sprays applied to previous crops), one can grow one's own delicious fresh parsley in one's kitchen in a sponge. By placing the sponge in a bowl with some water in the bottom, it may be kept continuously moist. Celery seeds and undoubtedly other seeds, as cress, etc., may be grown in the same way. With several dozen such bowls and sponges in one's kitchen producing different plants, one can have a "home-grown" supply of safe, unpoisoned sources of vitamins and minerals to replace the contaminated products on the market.

Be sure the seeds and legumes you use for sprouting have been organically grown, since seeds can transmit chemical fertilizer and spray residues from the plant that bore them. Organically grown alfalfa seeds, imported Chinese mung beans, imported Portuguese chick peas, organically grown sunflower seeds, etc. are all now available.

Health Value of Turkish Organic Foods

The following is quoted from an article by Karekin B. Kalustyan, on Zaro Agha, long-lived Turk of Ripley "Believe It or Not" fame, who lived to be over one hundred and fifty years old on a diet which was both vegetarian and organically grown. (Many American vegetarians, who live on chemically fertilized, sprayed foods, live no longer than conventional eater, and often they die sooner as a result of chronic spray poisoning. Zora, however, lived all his life on foods grown without chemical fertilizers or sprays, which are not generally employed in Turkey.

Mr. Kalustyan, who comes from Turkey, says that he has seen Zaro many times in Istanbul, Turkey, where he lived. He reports that Zaro's answer to the question about the secret of his longevity was: "Eat simple foods as Nature prepares them. Don't smoke or drink. Live entirely on the products of the soil, which are the basic elements of life."

During his long lifetime, Zaro lived mostly on the following foods: (1) Sun-dried black olives and onions, (2) Halva (made of Tahini, or Turkish sesame seed cream with organic Turkish grape butter, a concentrate of pure grape juice),

(3) Walnuts and filberts with raisins, (4) Fresh Romaine lettuce with yoghurt, made from sheep's milk, (5) Watermelon or honeydew melon with sheep's cheese, (6) Fresh organically grown apricaots with sheep's cheese, (7) Sheep's milk yogurt mixed with grape juice, (8) Organically grown raisins heated in water, with small pieces of whole wheat bread cooked, with virgin sesame seed oil added upon cooling, (10) Goat's or sheep's cheese and organic grapes, (11) Cracked wheat with pure butter, home-churned, and cooked organically grown tomatoes with wholewheat bread made from stone-ground wholewheat flour, and baked at home in a fire pit.

Zaro ate plenty of organically grown cucumbers and melons. His diet list excludes cow's meat or pork, fowl, fish and eggs. Also he used no cow's milk or dairy products. It is remarkable that the Hunzas, the long-lived disease-free race of the Himalayas, also avoid use of these same foods and live on a diet similar to Zaro's.

Zaro, also, besides avoiding foods grown with chemicals, used no chemically treated drinking water, but only pure spring water. As a beverage he used a mixture of 70% goat or sheep's milk yogurt or the same percentage of Grape Nectar with water.

It was Zaro's living example that converted Mr. Kalustyan, who was once a heavy smoker and conncumer of alsohol and strong coffee. Mr. Kalustyan then gave up these vices and reformed his way of living. He writes: "Having in view the life of Zaro, I, who was a heavy chain-smoker and consumer of alcohol and strong Turkish coffee, revised my way of life and found my health, and at seventy I am much healthier than my four brothers, all younger than myself. As a retired minister of the Seventh Day Adventist Church, on seeing in this country how peddlers of artificial vitamins are taking advantage of the people, I decided to aid my fellows who share my philosophy of life by procuring and supplying them with unexcelled organic foods of my mother country and its neighbors, where foods are not grown with artificial fertilizers and chemical sprays, the only method of fertilization being the rotation of crops and use of animal manure or rotten hay."

When asked how foods were grown in his own country, and whether chemical fertilizers and poisonous sprays are employed in the growing of Turkish foods, the brother of Mr. Kalustyan replied: "We Turks are too poor to afford such American luxuries. Turkish foods are grown without chemical fertilizers or sprays, nor are they fumigated, as practically all American foods are."

For this reason Turkish sesame seeds and products (halva, tahini, etc.) are better than domestic sesame seeds grown with chemicals. Turkish lentils and butter beans are better than American legumes. Turkish nuts and dried fruits (raisins, dates and figs) are better than those grown in this country, which are chemically fertilized, sprays, often bleached, sulphured and fumigated, and the same applies to Turkish fruit concentrates, nectars and butters, all of which products are imported into this country by Mr. Kalustyan's brother, an importer in New York, and distributed by Organic Food Research Associates, 215 Sixth Street, Lorain, Ohio.

Lentils, A Perfect Meat Substitute

Of all members of the vegetable kingdom, the lentil is unique in its capacity to serve as a meat substitute, and that is why we recommend to use cooked mashed lentils as a base for a sunflower seed meat loaf, mixing with other ingredients, and then baking or preparing as patties. The reasons why lentils possess to such a high degree the qualifications to serve as the base of a meat substitue are the following: (1) Their deep reddish-brown color resembles meat, so that lentil meat substances look like meat, (2) Their protein content is exceptional in its similarity to meat protein, (3) Like meat they contain iron, more so than other legumes and most other foods, (4) When properly prepared, with sunflower seed, sesame seed and pepitoria squash seed meal, under the influence of high temperatures during baking or frying, lentils, prepared as a meat substitute, have a remarkable meat-like taste.

The lentil has been a staple food in Egypt for thousands of years and is still a chief protein food of the Egyptians. A red Egyptian split lentil is available in this country, which, like split peas, is skinless with each half separated. It is remarkable because of the speed with which it cooks, taking only a short time to be ready; and since it readily turns into a puree, it is excellent as a base for soups, and can also serve to make lentil-sunflower seed-sesame seed meat substitutes. This red split lentil is rich in iron; and, being imported from Turkey, where agriculture is more natural, it is to be preferred to chemically fertilized (and possibly sprayed) American legumes. There is also a green onion-skin quick-cooking lentil imported from Turkey; and a larger brown South American lentil is also available, which has a very meaty flavor when made into meat substitutes. In general, the lentil is superior to the soy bean as the base of meat substitutes that look and taste like meat, even though the soy bean is richer in protein. The green Turkish lentil or the large brown South American are best for making meat substitutes.

According to the view that it is the extractives of meat that give it its flavor, these being chiefly purin bodies, lentils contain these. According to Besseau, while lentils have 5cg. purin bodies in 100 grams, peas have only 1.8cg. Nevertheless lentils are more easily digested than beans, whose excessive sulphur content causes them to produce flatulence.

In spite of the fact that legumes, including beans, peas and lentils contain pruins, they also are high in alkaline minerals, which neutralize and counteract pruins, whereas, on the other hand, foods such as meat, eggs, wheat and nuts, whose reaction is more acid, lack this capacity. Kellogg says that although all legumes contain purin bodies which are converted into uric acid, the amount is small as compared with that contained in meat. Dried beans contain only four grains of uric acid to the pound, whereas dried beans contain 56 grains. Kellogg considers lentil protein as superior to pea protein, and pea protein superior to bean protein.

Lorand syas that the best way to use lentils is as a puree, since it is the retention of the skin over the legume that causes retention of undigested fragments, which is the main reason why legumes often disagree. When lentils are mashed in the manner suggested below for making a meat substitute, this difficulty is overcome.

Strumpel found that when lentils are soaked and then cooked, about 40 per cent of the protein is unassimilated, whereas when prepared as a puree only 9 per cent is lost; and the same relation holds good in the case of beans. Also purees of lentils, beans and peas have less tendency to cause putrefaction and autointoxication than when these are eaten whole. Those with weak digestions are advised to use legumes only in this form. Still another way to use legumes is to prepare them in a soup and use only the dissolved mineral extract while discarding solid protein residue.

Lentils are particularly valuable because of their richness in iron; and are one of the few vegetable proteins that can replace meat protein, while at the same place supplying so much iron. From viewpoint of eye appeal, a lentil meat loaf has much the appearance of meat. The lentil has as much iron as egg yold. Beans and peas also have much iron. Except for for the soy bean, the biological value of lentil protein is higher than that of all other legumes, as is also its lecithin content. Lorand says: "That lentils are so neglected as never to be included in the bill of fare in the incomprehensible anomalies too often met with in the present-day scheme of staple food, used in place of meat. In many ways it surpasses the soy bean, which is overrich in protein and tends to strain the kidneys. (Experiments have shown that high protein soybean diets cause kidney degeneration just as high protein meat diets do.

How to Make a Lentil Meat Loaf

To prepare lentil meat substitutes that look and taste like meat, lentils should first be soaked and then cooked in glass-distilled water, after which they should be mashed, and then mixed with sunflower seed meal, with or without sesame seed and pepitoria seed meals. Add sage, majorum or basil, also onions, tomatoes and other ingredients of a vegetable meat loaf., which is then baked, after which the loaf may be sliced and prepared as patties, and served dressed with a tomato sauce. Such a lentil meat loaf will look and taste like meat, but is far more healthful than meat and does not tend to putrefy and cause constipation and autointoxication as meat does.

Chick Peas (Garbanzos), a Valuable Alkaline Food

The chick pea, due to its low protein content and high alkalinity, is non-uric-acid-forming and does not tend to introduce purins into the body. Therefore, those who suffer from uric acid conditions will do well to prefer chick peas to other legumes and protein foods, and of course to avoid meats entirely. And since green beans in the shell are more alkaline and lower in protein than the dried ones (their carbohydrates turning into protein during the process of maturing), it is clear that green beans have less tendency to introduce purin bodies into the system, and should be preferred.

The chick pea is undoubtedly one of the most healthful of all legumes, which is widely used throughout the world, and is not especially a Spanish food, as generally believed. It is widely used in India, in Turkey and other countries of the Near East, and throughout Cnetral and South America.

Due to its lower protein content, it is more digestible than most other legumes and is less gas-producing, especially when its skin is removed, which may be readily done by first soaking overnight and then rubbing with ahses, after which they are washed. This is the method employed by the Maya Indians. It increases digestibility by elimination of the skin and decreases cooking time. They then make the base for an excellent soup, or may be cooked and eaten with wild rice or millet.

Be sure to soak and cook chick peas and other foods with glass-distilled water, and never with hard water, which makes them tougher and take longer to cook. Glass-distilled water is also better for health. Cook only in glass.

Toasted chick peas are a favorite food in Mexico and the Near East. They are available in two forms, with and without skins. The skinless toasted chick peas are very tender and crunchy and provide a rich source of high quality proteins, magnesium and other minerals. An excellent way to prepare toasted chick peas is to first soak them overnight and then place on a baking pan in the oven, carefully regulating the temperature. When properly toasted, they are most delicious and quite tender.

We shall explain below how to sprout chick peas. Without doubt, they are best used in the sprouted form. It is best to sprout all chick peas before cooking, as this greatly reduces cooking time and increases their vitamin value.

The Basques, a mountainous folk of North Spain, who are noted for their tall stature and superior health and vigor, like the Hunzas of the Himalayas, use chick peas as a basic protein in their diet, in place of meat. (The Hunzas are practically vegetarians who eat meat only occasionally and not as a steady part of their diet, which consists chiefly of millet, chick peas, vegetables, apricots, etc.)

A comparison of the chick pea and the soy beans shows that the former is a much more desirable and more digestible food, especially when its skin is removed prior to cooking. Due to its low protein content (about 14% and its high content of magnesium and other alkaline minerals, the chick pea has a definite alkaline effect on the system and is much easier to digest and handle than the excessively protein-rich soy bean. The digestibility of both these legumes is furthermore increased when used in sprouted form; they then become richer in vitamins and more alkaline.

Toasted chick pea meal is used in Turkey. It is very nutritious and can be eaten as ir or mixed with other foods.

There are two main types of chich pea available in this country, the Mexican and the Portuguese. The latter represents a superior quality chick pea, with superior flavor and value. Tests have shown that when Mexican chick peas failed to sprout, the Portuguese did, indicating greater vitality. They are generally preferred because of their better flavor.

Chick peas, due to their low protein content and high alkalinity, do not form uric acid in the system as certain other purin-containing legumes do. They are one of the most healthful of all legumes.

Millet, Alkaline Super Grain

Millet is a true Organic Super Food worthy of universal use. Yet unfortunately, its superior nutritional qualities are practically unknown to people in this country; and except for a small minority of health-minded people, millet is not consumed in America except by the bird population. On the other hand, an inferior grain, wheat, is the one in general use.

But more "backward" races seem wiser, for among the Chinese, Hindue and peoples of the Near East, millet is in common use, as it also is in Africa. While it is generally believed that the Chinese live on rice, millet is the basic grain of most of China, especially in the northern parts where it is too cold to grow rice. It has been observed that the millet-eating North Chinese are far superior in physique to the rice-eating population of South China, indicating that millet, by its more alkaline reaction, has greater calcium-conserving capacity than rice.

Millet has the following nutritional virtues: 1. It is a very economical food - an ideal food for depression times. In fact it is one of the cheapest foods known, capable of supplying maximum and most balanced nourishment for its cost. Hence it proved a lifesaver for millions of Russians during the Russian famine, enabling them to keep in good health, whereas if wheat or any other acid-forming grain was used exclusively, as millet was at this time, they would have suffered from malnutrition (i.e., really demineralization produced by acidosis resulting from a one-sided, acid-forming diet). An example of the virtue of millet as an economical food was furnished by a poor family, without work or income, which settled in South Florida. Having been vegetarians and hearing about the value of millet, and having only a few dollars, they decided to invest this money to buy a hundred pound bag of hulled millet. For about a year the entire family, consisting of two adults and three children, lived largely on this bag of millet. Since millet on cooking, swells to many times its original size, only a few penniew worth sufficed to provide the family with all they could eat each day; and since it is such a well balanced, alkaline and nutritious food, millet satisfied them more than if they had lived on a variety of acid-forming foods. In evidence of the superior virtues of millet as an economical and at the same time a highly nutritious and healthful food, it may be noted that the millet diet kept these two adults and three children in good health furing this period, as well as solved an economic problem they would otherwise have been unable to solve. However, this idea of living on millet was not original with the, since millions of poor Orientals and Africans have done the same thing for centuries and for thousands of years, back to the days of Pythagoras, who, 2500 years ago, highly praised the nutritional value of millet, which was at that time already an ancient food, consumed by the Egyptians for thousands of years previously. It is interesting to note that Pythagoras himself, who advocated a low protein vegetarian diet, which his followers adopted, used millet and sesame seeds as the basic carbohydrate and protein food in his diet.

2. Millet is non-fattening, due undoubtedly to its alkaline tendency, since alkalies tend to dissolve and counteract fat formation. On the other hand, wheat is believed to form fat rather than muscle.

3. Due to its alkaline properties and its freedom from coarse, irritating bran, as well as due to the bland, soothing mucilaginous substance it gives off when cooked, millet is one of the easiest of all grains to digest, even by the tenderest stomachs and therefore to be recommended to persons suffering from dyspepsia, acid indigestion, gastro-intestinal inflammation, ulceration, etc., as for those suffering from acidosis and who are allergic to wheat for this reason.

4. Millet is richer in vitamins and minerals than other grains, except wild rice. It is quite rich in vitamin B complex; and, according to the researches of Profs. Osborne and Mendel, it contains all essential vitamins, as well as all minerals.

5. Osborne and Mendel found also that millet is unique among grains not only because of its completeness in vitamin content, but also because it contains all essential amino acids, and therefore it furnisheds a "complete" protein, whereas the proteins of other grains are incomplete and therefore unable to sustain animals in health.

6. Millet, as noted, is the only alkaline grain, and therefore valuable for sufferers from acid conditions, as rheumatism, arthritis, diabetes, etc., who would do well to avoid wheat in all forms due to its uric-acid-forming tendency, uric acid being a major contributory factor in these and other diseases.

7. Millet is definitely laxative, yet without the irritating and harmful effect of bran. The mucilaginous substance it gives off acts as an intestinal lubricant and aids elimination.

8. Millet is undoubtedly the tastiest of all grains, having an egg-yolk-like taste which may lead one to believe it has a high lecithin content. (Being related to corn, which is rich in fat-containing lecithin, the lecithin content of millet is higher than that of most other grains.) Millet is practically the only grain which is flavorful when eaten by itself without addition of salt or fat, which is not true of wheat and rye, which are flat and insipid when so prepared. This is undoubtedly due to millet's higher mineral content. Those who are anxious to go on salt-free diets and who find other cereals tasteless without salt, will, for this reason do well to use millet instead.

Millet, which is one of the oldest foods of the human race, is still a basic nutriment for millions in Asia and Africa, many of whose inhabitants live largely or even exclusively on it, when other foods are not available. The capacity of millet to support life, when used as an exclusive food, as mentioned above, was proven during the Russian famine, when it saved the lives of millions of people from starvation. The capacity of an exclusive millet diet to support life in good health, whereas if other acid-forming, more one-sided grains were used, disease and death would occur from progressive demineralization and vitamin deficiency. This was clearly demonstrated by the experiments of Osborne and Mendel at Yale University. They fed animals on diets composed exclusively of various grains to compare their effects. In the case of the acid-forming grains, as wheat, rue and oats, the animals developed acidosis, leading to vitamin and mineral deficiency, got sick and died.

Millet was the only grain tested that was found able to maintain animals in good health. The experimenters concluded that millet contains a nutritional balance of all elements essential for life - including the necessary amino acids (complete proteins), fats (including lecithin and other phosphatides), unsaturated fatty acids, carbohydrates, minerals and vitamins. This explains the capacity of races in various parts of the world to live almost entirely on this food and remain in good health. Due to its alkaline properties, millet does not cause mineral withdrawal and decalcification as the acid-forming grains, like wheat and oats, do.

In view of these facts, it is clear that millet should provide the base for an excellent therapeutic mono diet, and be better than rice, as employed in the rice-and-distilled water should be better than one of rice and distilled water from the viewpoint of mineral conservation. The therapeutic possibilities of a millet Organic Mono Diet, which is made tastier and more complete by addition of sesame seed meal and Japanese sea vegetation to the millet, should be carefully studied, especially for the treatment of persons suffering ill effects from the use of chemically fertilized vegetables sprayed with DDT, chlordane and other poisonous insecticides, whose residues they contain.

How to Prepare Millet

First secure organically grown hulled millet. It is easier to secure organically grown millet than other grains, since millet is not so apt to be grown with chemical fertilizers or sprays, since it grows well even on comparatively poor soil. It is also possible to secure millet that has not been fumigated with poisons as wheat and other grain crops have been. One of the largest millet growers in this country, who produces millet for human consumption, which he hulls, offers hulled millet grown without chemicals and unfumigated.

Do not try to cook unhulled millet, or bird seed, as the hull is too hard to cook. If you wish to use the entire millet seed, buy millet meal or flour and prepare it as a cereal or use in baking. A delicious unleavened alkaline millet bread can be made, alone or mixed with white or yellow cornmeal, or both, adding some grated fresh coconut, seed meal or fine hempseed meal. (Follow the same recipe as recommended above for making an unleavened corn bread.)

Do not be afraid that the hulling of millet removes its nutrients, for it does not. They are present in hulled millet as they are in hulled sesame seeds. All that is removed by the hulling process is the hard outer shell of millet, not its or vitamins.

There are many varieties of millet, most of which are grown chiefly as forage crops and not for human consumption. A variety of millet known as "Proso" is generally grown in Russia as a human food and constitutes a basic part of the Russian diet. Proso millet, sometimes called "proso" has been introduced into this country and is grown extensively in North Dakota, where much of the millet is grown without the use of chemical fertilizers or sprays.

To prepare millet, it may be cooked toasted or untoasted. The Russian method is to first shake the millet grains over a hot frying pan until they become crisp, or they may be placed on a baking pan in the oven until thoroughly dry. This toasting process improves flavor and reduces cooking time. Another way to reduce cooking time is to soak the millet overnight before cooking. (By this simple practice, the cooking time of all grains and legumes may be reduced and their vitamin value correspondingly increased.)

Be sure to use only glass-distilled water and glass untensils in preparing millet. It is best to use a glass double boiler if you cook over the flame. Use five parts of water to one part of millet, and add one part of sesame seed meal to gove a delicious fatty flavor. Then no further fat need be added to millet when eaten. Sesame seed meal is much better than cholesterol-containing butter. Cornmeal may be similarly prepared with sesame seed meal.

If you do not have a double boiler, you may cook millet over a flame in a glass casserole or pot, but be sure to place an asbestos pad between the flame and the pot and carefully regualte the flame after the water starts to boul, turning it down as low as possible, thereby avoiding the danger of the millet sticking to the bottom of the pot, which is the chief cause of the breakage of glass cookware.

The easiest and surest way to prepare millet is to add one part of millet, five parts of water and one part of sesame seed meal, flaxseed meal, fine hempseed meal or pepitoria squash seed meal to a glass baking casserole, cover and put in an oven for about three quarters of an hour. Since the heat is equally distributed there is no danger of the millet sticking to the bottom fo the casserole. The millet can then be eaten as a hot cereal or put in a cool place and left to congeal, whereupon it may be sliced, and prepared as patties with virgin sesame seed oil (the most digestible oil for frying, except natural, unrefined coconut oil. Or the slices cf the congealed millet may be dipped in virgin sesame seed oil or sesame seed meal and baked crisp in the oven, and eaten as an alkaline, non-fattening substitute for acid-forming wheat bread.

Wild Rice

Vitamin-Rich Seed of a Wild Grass

Nutritional Superiority of Wild Rice Over Acid-forming, Decalcifying Grains: Wheat, Rye and Oats

Wild rice is a true Organic Super Food whose remarkable nutritional value few people realize. Nor are they aware of the fact that in spite of its higher price, it is worth every cent paid for it-for it is so rich in vitamins and other nutrients, and has such healthful qualities in general, that one really obtains more, in real nutrition and vitamins, for every cent paid for wild rice than for the purchase of other cheaper and inferior grains. In fact, as Prof. McCollum and other nutritionists have pointed out, most grains not only fail to add minerals to the body, but actually, by their acid effects, rob minerals, especially calcium. McCollum therefore considers grain-eating a cause of tooth deterioration, pointing to the inhabitants of the Islands of Aran, off the coast of Scotland, who eat no grain whatsoever, using potatoes instead, and who have perfect teeth. So surely the cost of wild rice, which does not have the demineralizing effect of other grains, but which, instead, supplies valuable minerals as well as vitamins, to the body, and which is free from the acid-forming, demineralizing and decalcifying effect of wheat, rye, oats and other grains (as demonstrated by Mellanby, whose experiments we shall describe later), is no more than the cost of dental care as results from eating these cheaper and less wholesome grains. Those who value their health will be willing to spend on wild rice - nature's vitamin capsule - the same money that others spend on dentists, doctors and vitamins. For wild rice provides both food and vitamins at the same time, and in a most delicious form. Wild rice, like millet, is unique in being a non-acid-forming grain, and therefore it does not rob calcium from the body as the acid-forming grains, as wheat do. Persons who suffer from calcium deficiency will do well to use it in place of wheat and rye, and then they will not have to use large amounts of milk and cheese to obtain calcium, as most wheat eaters do-endeavoring to replace the calcium which wheat withdraws, but unfortunately taking in an excess of harmful cholesterol to the bargain.

Much better than taking that chemically contaminated product known as "bread", is to take a dish of wild rice. Wild rice supplies valuable minerals and vitamins, whereas ordinary bread contains next to none, except a few synthetic additives. Wild rice has been grown by Nature without human interference and without chemical fertilizers and sprays, nor has it been fumigated, as the grain from which bread is made has been. Wild rice, properly prepared, is very delicious, highly digestible and counteracts acids in the system, rather than adds to them, as wheat does.

The great nutritive virtues of wild rice, today unknown to and disregarded by the American people, were highly appreciated by the American Indians, for whom it was a favorite food and on which they lived whenever it was available. Today, as during centuries past, the Indians still pick wild rice in their canoes, being careful to always drop some grains into the water, to be assured of a crop the following year. For unlike ordinary rice, which is chemically fertilized, wild rice, which is a water plant, is one of the few foods on the market which has never been contaminated with chemicals. This is impossible, since it grows in the water.

This seed of wild grass has all the vitamin-and mineral-richness of grass concentrated in its seed, where Nature stores the finest elements of the plant, for the support of the growth of the young seedling. When soaked overnight, wild rice swells to many times its volume, and the grains open up, giving off a delightful aroma suggesting newly mown hay. (On the other hand, soaked brown rice is odorless. This is indicative of the superior vitamin-richness of this seed of a wild grass, when compared with rice. While rice is acid in reaction, wild rice is alkaline.)

HOW TO PREPARE WILD RICE

Wild rice should be purchased in cases of a dozen boxes, thereby securing advantage of a lower wholesale price. This will be one of the best investments in health that one can make. Do not contaminate this wonderful Organic Super Food by cooking it with chlorinated, metallized and flouridated city water, but use only glass-distilled water. Also do not use a metallic or enamelled cooking utensil, but cook it in a glass double boiler.

Wild rice should first be washed by several rinsings of water to remove its bitterish taste, and then should be soaked overnight in glass-distilled water, being careful to add sufficient water, since the rice increases greatly in volume while soaking. Use four times as much water as rice, though the soaked rice will require a little less. Add some dried Japanese sea vegetation, after prior washing and soaking.

Another excellent way to prepare wild rice is to first soak the rice overnight and then add to a glass baking casserole with four parts of water, sesame seed meal, Japanese sea vegetation, herbs, etc. and place in the oven, with casserole covered, until done. This is better than cooking over a direct flame, when there is danger of the rice sticking to the bottom and burning, unless an asbestos pad is used and a small flame, or else a double boiler.

If organically grown onions, tomatoes, celery, etc. are available, wild rice is delicious served with a tomato sauce, also with mung bean sprouts stewed in virgin sesame seed oil with onions and celery, in chop suey style. Such a dish provides a healthful, delicious low protein meal.

Wild rice, being a complete and balanced food, can be eaten at each meal, without tiring. It is the vitamin and mineral deficiencies of foods that makes one tire of them and crave others to overcome their deficiencies, but wild rice, used as the base of an Organic Mono Diet, proves perfectly satisfactory and keeps one in perfect health, and with a feeling of nutritional repletion after each meal. Brown rice, on the other hand, is an incomplete food and is only satisfactory together with other foods, whereas wild rice can be eaten as the base of a meal, being complete in itself.

How To Season Foods Without Using Salt or Other Harmful Condiments

By addition of various Japanese sea plant, as well as organically grown culinary hervs, to one's foods, they may be given a delicious flavor, as well higher vitamin vitamin value, without having to use salt or other harmful condiments, as pepper, etc. The art of seasoning foods with culinary herbs has been lost to the modern world. Growing wild or more naturally than chemically fertilized market vegetables, these herbs are more apt to contain trace minerals and rarer elements absent from ordinary foods; and it is for this reason that most of the culinary herbs, as sage and others, for centuries have been used as medicines, as well as for seasoning purposes.

Do not compare culinary herbs with spices. While the latter are more or less irritating to the gastro-intestinal mucous lining, and harmful, culinary herbs are beneficial and harmless, while at the same time giving foods a delicious flavor. By making foods more appetizing, they increase the flow of digestive juices and so help digestion.

Culinary herbs should best be used in combination with sea vegetation, such as Irish sea lettuce (leaf dulse) and Japanese sea plants, which, being rich in organic sodium chloride, supply foods with this substance, to appease the craving for salt. Sea vegetation, like culinary herbs, besides giving flavor to foods, enriches them with vitamins and trace minerals in abundance.

While the general recommendation is to use culinary herbs sparingly, since an excess undoes its won effect, in view of the richness of culinary Herbs in vitamins and minerals which most foods lack, the writer believes it advantageous to add them liberally, and later, at the end of cooking, to add a small amount for seasoning purposes, preferably after the heat has been turned and the food still hot and covered.

Therapeutic Value of an Organic Mono Diet

The wild rice-sesame seed-sea vegetation combination above described provides the base for a balanced, nutritious, therapeutic Organic Mono Diet, of value to persons who have suffered from chemical fertilizer and spray poisoning from use of ordinary vegetables and fruits, or from poisoning by uric acid and other organic toxins introduced by a high protein diet containing meat, foul fish and eggs, with its usual after-effects of constipation and autointoxication

The wild rice combination has been experimentally tried by the writer for over a year, during which time he ate no chemically fertilized, sprayed produce from the general market, and it proved highly successful as a basic diet, supplying MORE, rather than less, vitamins and minerals than ordinary vegetables and without any ill effects. The foods were cooked with glass-distilled water in a glass cooking utensil or baked in a glass casserole. After eating wild ric for some time, all other grains seemed relatively valueless and insipid; and he found it to surpass even millet. If fact, in evidence of the nutritional completeness of wild rice, the longer it was used, the more delicious it tasted, which is in marked contrast to other one-sided foods, which, under such conditions become monotonous and even repulsive.

This Organic Mono Diet is better than a complete fast, since it keeps the body well nourished, prevents undue loss of weitht, and at the same time remineralizes and revitaminizes, without adding anything objectionable. Meanwhile, it helps the body elimiate the toxic residues of previous foods, including chemical fertilezer and spray toxins, organic acid toxins from rich protein foods, etc. Both the vegetarian and the non-vegetarian will be beneficed by this wild rice Mono Diet. However it would be a mistake to attempt to live on wild rice and distilled water alone, without adding some or all of the ingredients mentioned, provided organically grown, such as sesame seed meal (or pine nut meal may be substituted), leaf dulse or Japanese sea vegetarian, and some mung bean sprouts stewed in virgin sesame seed oil, spread over the wild rice. Also use organically grown culinary herbs for seasoning. If wild rice is not available, use millet instead and prepare in the same way. Such a regimen will produce similar effects as the rice and distilled water diet used for heart conditions and the grain and distilled water diet employed for cancer. However, since it is nutritionally more complete, more satisfying and tastier, it can be prolonged for a much longer time, in fact, continued indefinitely; and surely this will be better than to live on too strict a diet of rice and distilled water for a short time, and then get tired of it and return to the use of the same foods than brought on the original illness. We may note in passing that plenty of coconut water shouldbe taken while on the wild rice mono diet. From the coconut meat, as explained before, a delicious cream may be derived which may be added to the wild rice while cooking, or coconut mild (coconut water plus cream) may be used for cooking the wild rice in place of distilled water. Fresh coconut oil, made from the coconut in the manner already described, is excellent as a fat to season the wild rice.

Every person who does not feel well should try such an Organic Mono Diet; and the writer is convinced that they will be delighted with the wonderful results they will derive therefrom, results certainly not obtainable when using chemically fertilized, sprayed vegetables and fruits purchased in public markets, or uric-acid-froming meat, fowl, fish, eggs or cheese.

Chapter Nine

THE ACID-BASE BALANCE

How It Determines Health or Disease

To eat only organically grown foods is not enough. Organically grown foods may be good or bad. They are bad when they are too acid-forming and produce acidosis. They are good when they maintain a healthful degree of alkalinity in the system. Some organically grown, or organic, foods are highly acid-forming and cause disease. Others are quite alkaline-forming and preserve and help maintain health. As important as it is to consume only organically grown foods, it is equally important to know how to balance your diet, so that it is predominantly alkaline, and protects you against acidosis and its resulting evils, which include vitamin and mineral deficiency.

One day we were visited by an organic farmer. Her lived entirely on organically grown foods he grew. He ate no chemically fertilized, sprayed products from the market, no white bread, nothing that was considered outside the category of organic foods. Yet he was not well. He was suffering from a rheumatic condition. He asked us why, living as he did on organically grown foods, he did not enjoy perfect health.

We inquired and discovered that though he ate only organic foods, his diet was highly acid-forming. The foods he ate produced considerable uric acid caused his rheumatic condition. The uric-acid-forming foods he ate that were responsible for his troubles were meat and whole wheat. His diet was unbalanced and was excessively acid-forming, with the result that his acid-base balance was upset, and shifted too much in the acid direction.

We advised him to change his diet, to cut out the acid-forming foods that were causing his illness and to live on an alkaline diet composed of alkaline-forming foods, as potatoes, vegetables, etc. We told him that he should use plenty of organically grown potatoes, since there is no food that is more alkaline and has greater capacity to neutralize uric acid and help him overcome his acid condition, which was the cause of his trouble.

Acid-Forming and Alkaline Forming Elements in Foods

Some forty years ago, Professor Sherman at Columbia University was the first to study the acid forming and alkaline forming elements of foods. His method consisted in reducing various foods to an ash and testing the ash for its acid or alkaline reaction. In general, it was found that all meats, fish, fowl, eggs, most nuts, wheat and oats were acid forming foods, while potatoes, melons, vegetables, bananas and fruits were alkaline forming foods.

Other observers found that acid forming diets predisposed to acidosis and disease, while alkaline forming diets tended to heighten the alkali reserve, which is the body's protection against disease. Most people make the mistake people make the mistake to consume an excess of acid forming foods, in the form of meat, eggs, bread, sugar, coffee, tea, etc., thereby lowering their alkali reserve and paving the way for acidosis and disease.

The human blood, in a state of health, is slightly alkaline in reaction. In states of disease it turns more acid, though it is still slightly alkaline.

The moment the blood turns acid, death occurs. So we see that life and death, health and disease are fundamentally determined by the delicate balance which exists between the acidity and alkalinity of the blood.

Generally the degree of acidity of alkalinity of the system is determined by urine analysis. When acid-forming foods are eaten, the urine turns more acid, and when alkaline forming foods are consumed, it turns more alkaline. Dr. Hindhede found that following the eating of meat or whole wheat, the urine showed considerable uric acid, which formed a visible precipitate, but when potatoes were eaten, they caused the urine to become alkaline and neutralize the uric acid introduced by the meat and wheat, bringing it into solution and eliminating it.

Glatherwick at Yale University, some years ago, conducted a comparative study of the acid and alkaline effects of foods on the human body. Of all foods tested, he found none to be more alkaline than baked potatoes. The more thoroughly the potato was baked, the more alkaline he found it to be. The only other food which he found that could come near to the potato in alkalinity was the cantelope. Bananas also were quite alkaline. On the other hand, meat, fowl, fish, eggs, wheat, prunes, plums and cranberries were all found to be acid forming. In the light of Blatherwick's studies, there is no food that has greater capacity to neutralize acid toxins in the blood stream and so help the body overcome acidosis and the diseases for which it is responsible than potatoes.

In the light of these facts we can understand why herbivorous animals, which feed on alkaline-forming vegetable foods, have an alkaline urine, whereas carnivorous animals which feed on meat have an acid urine, and why vegetarians have an alkaline urine, whereas meat-eaters have an acid urine. McCollum found that when cows were fed on wheat or oats, even when they consumed the entire plant, their urines were acid, and they gave birth to sickly and stillborn calves, but when they fed on corn, plant and all, their urines were alkaline and they gave birth to viable and healthy calves. Also the corn-fed cows produced more and better milk than the wheat or oat fed ones, shose diet was more acid forming.

The Decalcifying Action of Grains: Wheat, Rye and Oats

That grains may rob calcium from the body has been definitely proven by the ecperiments of the eminent English nutritionist Mellanby, who found that certain grains, as wheat, rye and oats, contain what he calls "anticalcifying" substances, which combine with calcium and withdraw this element from the teeth and bones. Mellanby ascertained this fact during his studies on the dietary origin of rickets. He found that whole oats were the most decalcifying of all grains, while rice was the least. Whole wheat and whole rye he also found to be decalcifying, more so than the respective refined grains, which would indicate that the decalcifying substance was associated with their protein, rather than their starch content.

The researches of Dr. Haig in England confirmed those of Mellanby. He found that whole oatmeal was the most uric acid forming of all grains, and rice the least. Could the "anticalcifying" substance of Mellanby be uric acid, which combines with calcium, forming calcium urates, which settle in the joints, causing the symptoms of rheumatism and arthritis?

There is reason to believe that this is so. Otherwise why should the grains that Haig found to be the most uric acid forming, as oatmeal and whole wheat, also be found by Mellanby to be most decalcifying; and why should the grain that Haig found to be the least uric acid forming, rice, be found by Mellanby to be the least decalcifying? Obviously it must be the uric acid which the decalcifying grains introduce into the system that causes them to withdraw calcium, for which this acid has a strong affinity.

Writing about Mellanby's researches, Blunt and Cowan, in their "Ultraviolet Light and Vitamin D in Nutrition", write: "It was a great surprise to find that substances containing the most calcium and phosphorus (oatmeal and wheat germ) were the most rich producing of rickets, while those that contained the least mineral (white flour and rice) were the least detrimental. The effects of the different cereals, therefore, would not be explained on the basis of their calcium and phosphorus content."

The explanation is that cereals that contained the most protein (as oats and whole wheat) were the most injurious to the teeth, more so that refined cerials are not injurious to the teeth and bones, for they are. It simply means that the respective whole grains, with their higher protein content, were still more harmful. The only explanation is that the stronger acids formed as end-products of protein metabolism had greater tendency to rob calcium from the teeth than the milder carbonic acid which is the end-product of carbohydrate metabolism.

Meat contains four times the amount of acids found in cerials, so that as acid forming and decalcifying as cereals are, meat is much more so, and more injurious to the teeth. This upsets the common idea that cerial starch is the chief cause of tooth decay, and that by cutting out all starches and living largely on a starch free high protein diet, tooth decay may be prevented. As a matter of fact, meat, eggs and ol¹ cheese (containing salt, which is decalcifying) form stronger acids, and hence have greater power to remove calcium from the teeth and bones, than cereals.

Whole Wheat Found More Acid Forming than White Bread!

The biochemist Horvath of the University of Delaware found that whole wheat was many times more acid forming than white bread. The reason for this is that the protein of grain, in the course of its metabolism, is transformed into a number of very strong acids; phosphorus, sulphuric, nitric, phosphoric and uric, which remain as free acids in the bloodstream unless eliminated through the kidneys. However, the kidneys can eliminate only a fixed quantity of the acid end-products of protein metabolism daily, with the result that the excess remains in the blood as free acids, attacking the bones and teeth and dissolving their calcium. In the case of starch, the situation is different. A relatively mild acid, carbonic acid, is formed. This is readily reduced to carbon dioxide and iliminated through the lungs, while an excess is carbohydrates is deposited as fat. This may explain whole oats, which are richer in protein than other grains, was found by Mellanby to be the most decalcifying, whereas white rice, which has the least protein, as found to be the least.

Experimental animals fed on either white bread or whole wheat bread eventually die from demineralization caused by acidosis. An exclusive rye diet produces the same effects, accompanied, according to Mellanby, by spinal de-

degeneration caused by what he believes is a toxic substance in rye. Whereas exclusive diets of various acid-forming grains failed to support life, in the case of a millet diet, Osborne and Mendel found that it maintained animals in perfect health, indicating that millet contains a balance of all nutritional essentials. Being alkaline in reaction, it does not lead to acidosis.

Dr. P.H. Holst of the University of Oslo found in wheat a decalcifying substance which he called a "toxamin", which acted antagonistically to the deposition of calcium in the bones.

The famous biochemist Bunge pointed out that wheat contains an excess of sulphuric acid which tends to cause acidosis, and that a diet consisting too largely of cereals tends to be injurious. Kellogg claims that if wheat intake were reduced by one half and replaced by potatoes, a great improvement in health would occur (provided, of course, that the potatoes were organically grown). Holst and Frohlich found that guinea pigs readily developed scurvy when restricted to a diet of wheat bread and cereals, but when potatoes were used they reamined healthy. The failure of the potato crop, and the use of wheat instead, has frequently led to epicemics of scurvy in Ireland, Norway and the eastern part of the United States.

Dr. Haig found that the outer jusk of whole wheat contained a certain quantity of xanthin, which forms uric acid in the body. He therefore excludes whote wheat and oatmeal from his uric-acid-free diet. In place of these acid-forming grains, he recommends alkaline-forming potatoes. He advises not to give children wheat in any form due to its tendency to cause retention of uric acid, which is the cause of rheumatism, bronchitis, etc. Instead, potatoes, which neutralize and help remove uric acid, should be used. Dr. Haig writes:

"These cereals often tend decidedly to raise the acidity of the urine, and when taken in quantity, over a length of time, especially in cold weather, they may not only do this, but also diminish the alkalinity of the blood; hence they tend to cause some retention of uric acid in the body, and, acting with other causes, may even lead toward gout and rheumatism. Thus horses suffer considerably from rheumatism when both too much dry cereal and too little fresh vegetables. Arthritis, both in man and horses, can be treated by increasing and maintaining the alkalinity of the blood. This can be done by eating vegetables which contain alkali, such as potatoes, and by diminishing the protein diminishes the formation of acids in the body."

For this reason Haig found that whole wheat, which is high in protein, was the most acid-forming and the least easy to digest of all grains, except whole oats, while rice was the least acid-forming and the easiest to digest. Dr. Chakraberty, a Hindu physiologist, says: "The general idea that bread is good for all people is a patheitc misconception. It is good for a muscular laborer, who needs its carbohydrates for his energy, but rice is better."

Dr. Knight, in his _Physiological and Horticultural Papers_, writes: "Bread made from wheat, when taken in large quantities, has probably, more than any other article of food in use in this country, the effect of overloading the alimentary canal; and the general practice of French physicians points out the prevalence of diseases arising among their patients (from this cause)." Rosewarne, in his Science of Nutrition Simplified, says: "For a large proportion of the population, for whom bread must be literally the staff of life, it is, moreover, one of the principal contributory causes of feebleness and numerous forms of ill-health."

Froude objects to wheat because of its acid-forming tendency, and advises that it be replaced by potatoes, which are alkaline in reaction. He says: "Grains are considered acid-forming. That is, they are considered capable of producing acidosis, because they are low in antifermentic and antitoxic food salts. This makes the excessive use of one of the great causes of hardening of the arteries and premature aging."

Concerning the superiority of potatoes as the ideal starchy food in place of grains, Froude writes: "The general health will be greatly improved if it were generally substituted for bread and cereals. It is easily digested, very nutritious, and is not acid-forming as are the grains."

Does Wheat Cause Hardening of the Arteries?

Dr. Densmore, in his work, "How Nature Cures", and Dr. De Lacy Evans, in his book, "How to Prolong Life," both present arguments to prove that all wheat products are conducive to premature decrepitude, leading to hardening of the arteries. The probably results from the uric acid which wheat forms, which combines with calcium to form calcium urates, which settle along the walls of the arteries, in the joints, etc. Carrington therefore calls bread the "staff of death."

Dr. Sansum, at the Santa Barbara Metabolic Clinic, experimentally demonstrated that whole wheat produces hardening of the arteries. He fed different groups of rabbits on high protein diets of meat and of whole wheat, and in either case they died from hardening of the arteries. While whole wheat tends to interfere with normal calcification by withdrawing calcium from the bones, it produces excessive calcification of the arteries. The calcium which its acid end-products of metabolism dissolve from the bones obviously combines with the uric acid it forms, forming insoluble calcium urates which settle along the walls of the arteries.

A century ago, an English chemist names Rowbatham claimed exactly what Sansum recently demonstrated. He said that the habitual use of wheat caused hardening of the arteries and premature old age, both in men and animals (horses), resulting from the encrustation of calcareous deposits within them. Rowbatham wrote: "Bread (from wheat flour), when considered in reference to the amount of nutritious matter it contains, may with justice by called the staff of life; but in regard to the amount of calcareous matter it contains, we may with equal justice call it the staff of death."

Heroditus, the Greek historian, describing a visit of some Persian ambassadors to the long-lived Ethiopians, asked what the Persian king was accustomed to eat, and to what age the longest-lived Persians had been known to attain. The ambassadors replied that their king ate bread, and described the nature of wheat - adding that eighty years was the longest term of man's life among the Persians.

Therefore the Ethiopians remarked that it did not surprise them that the Persians had such short lives, and that "if they fed on dirt (the term used for wheat), that they died so soon."

Superiority of Rye Over Wheat

There can be no doubt that rye is far superior to wheat, which is more acid-forming and decalcifying because richer in protein and relatively poorer in minerals, its greater acidity accounting for the fact that it is more fattening than rye, whereas rye is better for the support of muscular activity. A comparison of the rickety and physically inferior English with the vigorous tall Russians who live on rye is evidence of this fact. Strong Russian laborers have been known to work hard all day on no other food than some black rye bread and some garlic. While wheat tends to promote fat formation, rye builds muscles, as shown by the example of rye-eating athletes. Rye-eating Finnish competitors walked away at the Olympic Games, with ten times their normal share of trophies when endurance was the test. A 66-year old Finnish bicycle rider won a 1000-mile race with 50 young contestants. His main item of diet sees to have been rye bread.

Rye forms less uric acid in the system than wheat or oats; and corn is still more alkaline, for while these other grains tend to turn the urine acid, McCollum found that corn turned it in the alkaline direction. Since acid intoxication of the muscular tissues, by accumulation of uric and other acids, is a chief cause of fatigue, we can understand why rye-eating races should surpass wheat-eating ones in endurance, since rye is richer in alkaline minerals and poorer in protein, therefore having less tendency to introduce uric acid into the body.

Superiority of Rice Over Rye and Wheat

Even better than rye is rice, for while, according to Haig, both wheat and rye are uric-acid-forming, rice is not. And since it is the accumulation of uric acid in the tissues that is a chief cause of muscular fatigue, we can understand why rice-eating Orientals have such indefatiguable energy and endurance, as compared with Occidental races that consume wheat and rye. The reamrkable capacity for hard labor possessed by Chinese Coolies and Japanese laborers who eat no other grain than rice, and whose diet is vegetarian and low in protein (and therefore is non-uric-acid-forming) is evidence of this fact.

Superiority of Millet Over Rice, Wheat and Rye

Much better than rice, however, is millet, for while rice is acid-forming (though not uric-acid-forming), millet is alkaline in reaction, and hence a better food for calcium retention, as indicated by the better developed bony structure of the millet-eating North Chinese in comparison with the rice-eating South Chinese, as previously mentioned.

It is strange that the American people should choose the most inferior of all grains - wheat - as their basic grain in place of the most superior of all grains - millet, which is practically unknown in this country, except for use as a bird food. While wheat is acid-forming and decalcifying, millet is alkaline in reaction and calcium-conserving, and while it is probably religious traditions, the old belief that wheat is the "staff of life", that is responsible for its universal use as a basic grain, in place of much superior grains, as buckwheat, barley, rice and millet, but with the advance of scientific knowledge of nutrition, more and more people will realize the inferiority of wheat as a food, and the superiority of millet.

Let us briefly review the reasons why millet is superior to wheat and realted acid-forming grains: (1) Millet is alkaline in reaction, while wheat in all forms is acid-forming, for which person, persons who suffer from acidosis and its various after-effects, as catarrhal conditions, colds, rheumatic symptons, hardening of the arteries, etc., will do well to use millet in place of wheat. (2) Millet is laxative without having the irritating effect of the rough bran of whole wheat, which, when eliminated and when whole wheat is converted into white flour, makes a pasty, constipating product. (3) Millet, due to its high alkalinity, is non-fattening, while wheat is definitely fattening, tending to form fat on the body, rather than muscle. (4) Millet is much tastier than wheat, due to its nutritional completeness, so that it can be eaten as is without addition of salt or fat, without which wheat is absolutely tasteless, all that are essential to life, and hence can prolong life indefinitely, whereas wheat lacks certain essential vitamins and minerals with the result that an exclusive wheat diet leads to malnutrition, disease and eventual death. (6) Millet contains all essential amino acids, and ther3fore provides a source of complete protein, whereas the proteins of wheat are incomplete. (7) Millet, since it grows in all climates of the world, is available to all races, whereas wheat is available to races only in certain cold climates, but not in warmer regions, unless shipped great distances. (8) Since millet is an easy crop to grow and produces on even poor land, being a soil enricher, there is less need to use chemical fertilizers on millet than on wheat, with resulting less need for spraying, so that millet is more likely to be grown naturally than wheat. (Organically grown millet, millet meal and millet flour are now available; and, incidentally, the largest supplier of hulled millet has grown it without chemicals not because of organic convictions, but simply because millet did not require any fertilizer, being one of the easiest crops to grow).

Bran a Harmful Food

Whole wheat, like whole rye, has another objection. Viewed under magnification, the bran of wheat looks quite frightening, especially when we bear in mind that this sharp, cutting, lacerating substance must pass through thirty feet of delicate mucous lining of the human intestinal tract. What possible damage this sharp, cutting substance must do to the soft mucous membrane, as it passes along, is worth considering. On this subject, Dr. Gibson writes: "The theory that bran is valuable as a laxative is based upon the same principle that a whip is a good tonic for a tired horse. The bran moves the bowels by sheer force of irritation - causing the injured tissues to exert a special effort to remove from the alimentary tract the offending agent. A similar effect is produced by sand or fine gravel...Furthermore, as the coarse hull of the grain begins to cause irritation of the lining of the stomach, the latter, as a means of self-protection, proceeds to floor the injured parts with secretions of hydrochloric acid, which in the course of time gives rise to an excess of acid in the system, with corresponding symptoms and neuralgic pains in the shoulders."

During a trip through Eastern Europe, the writer once tried eating the coarse, dark heavy whole rye bread so popular among the peasantry. While they have adapted their digestive organs to the irritating effect of its bran, the writer, coming from America where such bread is practically unknown and who was unaccustomed to such coarse fare, was not so adapted. On eating the heavy black rye bread, he found that it produced a state of intestinal inflammation manifesting in bloody stools. He had previously observed this after eating whole wheat bread for some time, which caused him to give up its use. In either case it was due to the irritating effect of bran.

In this connection, the following interesting case, which was reported to the writer, may be mentioned. A Russian peasant who, as is the rule, lived on coarse black rye bread as his basic food, suffered from a stomach ulcer which his doctor pronounced incurable. Then came the famine that followed in the wake of the first world war. He found himself without food. Searching in his barn he found some bags of millet which he had stored for his chickens which no longer existed. So he commenced to live on millet. For six months he ate nothing but millet. On this diet he felt in excellent health. At the end of this time he went to his doctor, wondering what effect his millet diet had on his ulcer. Much to the surprise of both the doctor and himself, it was found that the ulcer had completely disappeared.

There are two explanations of this. First of all, while the bran of whole rye has an irritating effect on the gastric lining and would therefore prevent the healing of ulcers, in the case of millet, it is just the opposite. While millet is laxative in its effects, it owes this property not to any irritating effect, since, when hulled (the only way in which it is suitable for human consumption), it is free from any coarse, irritating outer layer, or bran, yet has its entire nutrients, as do other grains in their unrefined form. When cooked, it exudes a mucilaginous substance, bearing some resemblence to the okrin of okra or the mucilaginous substance given off by sea vegetation, which has a definitely bland, soothing action on the gastrointestinal mucous lining. Secondly, whereas wheat and rye have an acid effect on the gastro-intestinal contents - and acidity is a factor in the aggravation of ulcer conditions - millet is unique among grains in being alkaline in reaction, and alkalinity is favorable for the healing of ulcers. Dr. Gernhardt at the Los Angeles Sanitarium fed patients on various grains and examined their urines. While whole wheat and rye produced acid urines, when millet was eaten, the urine turned alkaline. (McCollum performed similar experiments on cows. He found that whereas wheat and oats, plant and all, produced acid urines, corn, plant and all, turned the urine alkaline. In the former case, the cows bore sickly or dead calves, but in the latter case all calves were healthy.)

Cane Sugar (Sucrose), A Physiological Irritant

Sucrose, or cane sugar, irritates any tissue with which it comes into contact, and it makes no difference whether it is present in the form of white sugar, "raw" sugar, which is not raw, but a product of repeated reheatings during the refining process to which sugar is subjected. Sucrose not only irritates the mucous lining of the mouth, but also that of the stomach and intestines. This often causes serious injury. In an experiment with sugar in the stomach, a solution of 5.7 per cent produced reddening of the mucous membrane of the stomach and predisposes to gastritis. Cane and beet sugar, as well as sorghum are all irritants. Sherman states that sugar is an irritant to the stomahc, and Kellogg says that cane sugar (including blackstrap molasses) contributes to gastric catarrh, acidity, indigestion, stomach ulcer, etc.

It is a significant fact that while the human stomach produces enzymes to digest lactose (milk sugar) as well as fructose or levulose (fruit sugar), it can produce no enzyme to digest sucrose (cane sugar). This accounts for the incapacity of infants to handle cane sugar, while they can very well handle milk sugar or fruit sugar, such as banana sugar. It also explins why cane sugar tends to set up alcohol fermentation in the human stomach and is difficult to digest. (Does this not explain why those who give up alcohol often become candy addicts, thereby gratifying their craving for alcohol by the alcohol that cane sugar, by its fermentation, forms in the stomach? Any may not the craving for fermented bread, which is one of the hardest food habits to give up for one addicted to it, be due to the same cause - a form of vicarious alcoholic resulting from the alcoholic fermentation of bread when in contact with the hydrochloric acid of the stomach?)

How Sugar is Manufactured: Why Brown Sugar, "Raw" Sugar and Blackstrap Molasses Are Manufactured

It is a popular idea among food reformers that while white sugar is considered injurious to health and a tooth-destroyer, brown sugar, "raw" sugar (really not raw, but a product of repeted reboilings with lime, etc.) and blackstrap molasses are "natural" sugars and good. The following facts about the manufacture and refining of sugar will make this clear.

First the extracted juice of the sugar cane is pressed out by steam-heated rollers. It is then clarified by heating with lime, which destroys most of the vitamins. The devitamized clarified juice is then concentrated to a crystalline form by boiling under vacuum. After at least three repeated boilings and recrystallizations, the final batch of sugar crystals is obtained. The non-crystallized juice is then run off as molasses, while the crystallized portion is sold as "raw" sugar. It is really not "raw" at all, since it is a product of repeated boilings, and is a devitamized product. The same is true of the much-advertised blackstrap molasses, an inferior by-product of white sugar manufacture for which producers are seeking to secure a market through exaggerated advertising claims.

After sugar cane juice has been clarified of its suspended foreign matter, as cane fibers, dead insects, soil particles, etc., which is done by passing through a fine copper screen, it is then filtered through some charcoal which absorbs coloring matter. The resulting decolorized sugar is then sold as white sugar, while from the non-crystallized colored syrup than remains, various brownsugars are produced. The final residue from these brown sugars is blackstrap molasses.

All cane sugar, whether white, brown, "raw" or blackstrap molasaes, is an indigestible, acid-forming, demineralizing and decalcifying product, which should find no place on a hygienic diet. The common idea that while white sugar destroys the teeth (destroying them from within, not from without, by the action of the carbonic acid it forms, which combines with calcium, which is withdrawn from the teeth), brown sugar, "raw" sugar and blackstrap molasses are safe and do not injure the teeth is false. All these cane sugar products are acid-forming and decalcifying)i.e., calcium robbers).

Alkaline Unfiltered Organically Grown Maple Syrup
Versus Blackstrap Molasses and Honey

Most maple trees today are sprayed with DDT and other poisons to protect them from pests that denude them of their leaves, these spray residues eventually finding their way into the maple sap and maple syrup. For this reason it is important to use only organically grown maple syrup. It is also important to use only maple syrup that has not been <u>filtered</u>, as most on the market have been in order to clarify them. The filtering process removes valuable minerals from maple syrup which are important to balance the acid-forming effect of its sugar, and create a more alkaline product. Unfiltered maple syrup, for this reason contains considerable alkaline minerals, as calcium, magnesium, etc., which are absent from the filtered product, which is consequently more acid-forming. Unfiltered maple syrup is more alkaline and better for calcium retention than blackstrap molasses or honey, its mineral content vastly surpassing that of honey. While it is true that maple syrup contains sucrose, its high content of alkaline minerals prevent it from having the bad effects of cane sugar products, provided it has been organically grown, unfiltered and not prepared in kettles of inferior materials, as aluminum, copper, etc. which might cause metallic contamination of the syrup while heated therein. Undoubtedly a <u>raw</u> maple syrup, which has not been subjected to the usual prolonged heating treatment, if placed on the market, would command a premium price among progressive food reformers.

Is Honey Really a Healthful Food?

The popular idea that whereas white sugar is bad for health, honey is good, and whereas white sugar injures the teeth, honey does not, is quite erroneous. Honey is a product of nectar from flowers which has been acted on by formic acid from a bee's organism, and is relatively poor in minerals in comparison with the acid-forming tendency of its high sugar content, being a much more mineral-poor, acid-forming and decalcifying sweetening agent that unfiltered maple syrup. The writer has known of cases where misguided persons, giving up sugar, commenced to use honey liberally, believing that since it was a "natural" sweet, it was good for them, and could be eaten freely, even excessively, without ill effects. The result was that their teeth became decalcified even at a faster rate than when they used white sugar, which, knowing that it was bad, they would tend to use more sparingly.

In a certain instance the members of a family of vegetarians who produced honey and earned their living selling it, and who, consequently, used it in quantity, found that they teeth gradually wore away to their roots, which became abscessed and had to be removed. Honey, being very acid-forming forms large quantities of carbonic acid in the blood, without sufficient alkaline minerals to balance it and hold it in check from attacking the teeth and robbing them of calcium.

Page 149

For this reason, the free use of honey, like of other mineral-poor concentrated sweets, gradually destroys the teeth, especially if used excessively together with an otherwise acid-forming diet.

Use of honey by vegetarians is an anomaly, since honey is an animal food in the true sense of the word, just as cow's milk is. The cow eats grass and from it produces a mammary secretion called milk. The bee takes nectar from a flower and by adding to it formic acid produced by glands of its body (this formic acid being a sort of "insect milk" forms the product known as honey.

In addition to formic acid, honey contains manite acid, which interacts with protein, forming alcohol, ammonia and carbonic acid. Thus honey introduces three acids into the body - formic, manite and carbonic. This produces acid fermentation in the stomach, leading in some cases to milder or severer nervous intoxication and systemic poisoning. The old Norse, by soaking malt grain in solution of honey, amde an alcoholic beverage named "nyod" (mead).

Many honeys are toxic due to bees going to flowers with toxic elements in their nectar. This is especially true when bees are in the vicinity of trees or plants that have been sprayed with poisonous insecticides. In East Nepaul, bees turn pollen of the Rhododnedron flower into a honey that produces a state of stupor similar to that produced by opium.

Combined with starches, the sugar of honey sets up fermentation and gas production. The laxative virtue ascribed to honey has its basis in this very fermentation, since the body, as an act of self-preservation, eliminates through the bowels the toxins and ptomaines generated by the mixture of honey with food.

Dr. A.E. Gibson writes: "It is a common popular belief that honey is a legitimate sweet, and can be used with dietetic safety where other kinds of sugar are regarded as dangerous. Nothing is combination with other foodstuffs even more dangerous than ordinary white sugar."

Healthful Alkaline Sources of Natural Fruit Sugar

There are several excellent substitutes for honey and cane sugar which have been importe from the Near East. One of these is carob or St. John's bread. This is a long dry fruit which is availabe in powdered form or as a thick syrup resembling molasses. In either case there is present levulose, or fruit sugar, in combination with an abundance of alkaline minerals. This is one of the finest sweetening agents, since it is sufficiently rich in minerals to prevent its highly digestible fruit sugar content from having any aicd-forming or decalcifying effect.

Another sweetening agent now available is Grape Nectar and Butter imported from Turkey. These are made entirely from the juice of organically grown Turkish grapes, which has been concentrated down to a syrup or a butter consistency. These products supply pure grape sugar, one of the best of all sugars, in combination with iron and alkaline mine als, so that when used as a sweetening agent, there is no harmful, acid-forming or decalcifying effect, but rather, in addition to sugar, valuable minerals and vitamins of the grape are supplied in concentrated form.

Another good source of sugar is provided by unfumigated, organically grown dates, as imported from Turkey or grown in California. (Be sure the California dates you buy are unfumigated as well as organically grown, since many so-called organically grown dates have been fumigated with poisons). Turkish pitted dates, Date Nectar (concentrated syrup of date sugar) and Date Butter are now on the market. Organically grown unsulphured raisins, Turkish and California, may also be used, and also organically grown Turkish or California figs, as sources of high quality fruit sugar.

All these sugars are rich in minerals, alkaline in reaction, and non-decalcifying, and are much better than the commonly used inferior, devitamized blackstrap molasses or demineralizing honey.

Dr. Hindhede's Researches on the Physiological Advantages
of an Alkaline Low Protein Diet

Dr. M. Hindhede, eminent Danish nutritionist and director of the Hindhede Laboratory for Nutritional Research, established by the Danish government in Copenhagen, was formerly a medical man who directed his attention to nutrition, in which field he eventually became a world authority. For many years he conducted a careful scientific research on the protein requirement of amn, the results of which were subsequently published in his work, "Protein and Nutrition." Dr. Hindhede, after careful study, showed that there is a definite relation between high protein diets, acidosis and thus help the body to develop greater resistance to disease.

During the first world war, when Denmark was blockaded for two years, Dr. Hindhede was appointed food commissioner of his country; and was authorized by the givernment to arrange a diet for the nation, involving a population of three million people, in accordance with scientific principles. In considering the problem of the conservation of Denmark's food supply, Dr. Hindhede decided that to feed cattle and seine with potatoes and cereals that might be used for human consumption was wasteful, since it meant a loss of approximately 80% of the nutritional value of the foods consumed by the animals, as compared with the yield in the form of their flesh. This means that a given amount of potatoes and grains that were enough to feed 100 people would feed only 20 people when given to animals and transformed into their flesh. For this reason the potatoes and grains were reserved for the use of the people, and the stock of cattle and swine was reduced.

The people received a sufficiency of potatoes, whole rye bread, barley porridge, an abundance of green vegetables and some milk and butter. The diet was lacto-vegetarian, flesh foods and eggs having been eliminated. In consequence of this enforced alteration of the dietetic habits of the Danish people, the death rate dropped as much as 34 per cent, being as low as 10.4 per cent when the regime was in force for one year. The diet was continued during the two years of the blockade, and was discontinued after it was over, with the result that the death and disease rate suddenly jumped to their previous much high level soon after the return to "normal" eating, involving the consumption of meat and other foods rich in protein.

On the basis of this mass experiment in nutrition, involving three million men, women and children, Dr. Hindhede was convinced that their improved health and lowered death rate while on the low protein lacto-vegetarian diet was due to the avoidance of the harmful effects of meat-eating and alcohol-drinking during this period, and therefore concluded that "the principal cause of death lies in food and drink."

In an article, "The Effect of Food Restriction During War on Mortality in Copenhagen," which appeared in the Journal of the American Medical Association, Feb. 7, 1920, Dr. Hindhede described his experience in feeding the Danish nation on a meatless diet during two years of the blockade:

"As research had also shown that man can retain full vigor for a year or longer on a diet of potatoes and fat and for half a year or more on a diet of barley and fat, reliance was placed on our potatoes and the large crop, which was given to man and not to pigs, as heretofore, with the result that the pigs died of starvation, but the people received sufficient nutrition...Our principal foods were bran bread, barley porridge, potatoes, greens, milk and some butter. Pork production was very low...Beef was so costly that only the rich could afford to buy it in sufficient quantity. It is evident, then, that most of the population was living on a milk and vegetable diet."

"The Danish food regulation was the most interesting problem for me. It was a low protein experiment on a large scale, about 3,000,000 subjects being available. What was the result? What was the effect on the health of the people? What was the death rate?"

"Placing the average ratio of deaths for the period 1900 to 1916 at 100, the variation being between 93 and 107, during the year of severe regulation it fell to 66, a decrease of 34 per cent.

"This result was not a suprising one to me. Since 1895, when I began my experiments with a low protein diet (mostly vegetarina), I have been convinced that better physical donditions resulted from this standard of living. It may be said that _a vegetarian diet is a more healthful diet than the ordinary diet._ As a result of extensive studies in this field, I am convinced that overnutrition, the result of palatable meat dishes, is one of the most common causes of disease."

"There are good reasons for believing that a diet composed of meat, eggs and white bread - a common diet of the well-to-do is far from being a healthful diet. Even in the case of rats, a meat diet seems eventually to be harmful. Although rats can thrive quite well on a meat diet - which man cannot do - the young of meat-fed rats seldom survive."

Elsewhere, Dr. Hindhede writes: "For many years I have been convinced that common stomach troubles and intestinal disorders very often arise from putrefaction caused by putrefying animal protein, as these complaints disappear, like dew under the morning sun, on a low protein diet. Since my family and myself have adopted a low protein diet, we have never been troubled with these maladies, - neither do we ever fuffer from summer diarrhea. But with a return to a rich meat diet, for experimental purposes, I contract colic and diarrhea with mathematical certainty.

"Possibly, from long experience of exclusively vegetable foods, my intestines have lost the power of producing antitoxins, which must be present if the toxins of meat putrefaction are to be counteracted."

"Is it not possible that the absence from the organism of these toxins is the cause of the feeling of buoyancy and increased endurance of which one is so often sensible on a low protein diet."

"But I have not the time to dwell longer on this interesting and complicated point; so I will refer the reader to Prof. Combe's work on autointoxication of the intestines. It will help us to better understand this point if we bear in mind the way in which an egg or piece of meat will rot. Flour does not become putrid like this, even though it be left standing, while wet, for some time. When rich meat is eaten similar putrefaction goes on in the intestinal tract; if only a small proportion of vegetable food is eaten with the meat; and the terrible offensive odor of the excreta after a meat diet will give some idea of the nature of the putrefaction. The excreta after a bread and potato diet have no such odor if these foods have been thoroughly masticated."

"If an egg be infected with feces, and left for some time, it will produce beneath the skin of a rabbit, the animal will speedily die. But if the same experiment be tried with corn, no poisonous products are forthcoming. Even if we dissolve the starch from flour so that only the protein remains and submit it to the same test, we shall fail to obtain any poisonous products."

For some time the Meat Trust has financed propaganda in favor of a liberal consumption of meat to supply amino acids and protein. Due to this publicity, a high protein fad has taken root, both in the mind of the general public and the medical profession. The idea is being spread that lack of protein is dangerous and may lead to disease, while a high protein diet is beneficial and strengthening. Though this idea is widely accepted, it does not stand on any scientific basis, as the careful experiments and extended research of Dr. Hindhede, conducted in his nutrition laboratory in Copenhagen, have clearly demonstrated. These experiments have shown that the human body is by nature a low tolerance for protein, and that all protein consumed in excess of this small amount is injurious, straining the kidneys and other vital organs in an effort to excrete its toxic end-products lest they poison the body as a whole or settle in the form of uric acid deposits, in the joints and elsewhere, causing rheumatic and other symptoms. For as long as 300 days and up to nearly two years, Dr. Hindhede maintained working men on low protein diets whose only source of protein was derived from potatoes, which composed almost their exclusive diet. Yet in spite of the fact that the potato contains only about 2 per cent protein, which is about as much as is present in most vegetables and fruits, these men injoyed excellent health and vigor, and showed no evidence of failing to obtain sufficient protein. By careful nitrogen equilibrium tests conducted during this period, Dr. Hindhede showed that even on such a low protein diet of potatoes and oliomargarine,, they were securing all the protein that their bodies required or could handle; and that any additional protein intake would be an excess. And when we consider the fact that most people ordinarily consume from 10 to 20 times more protein than did these men on potato diets, and that this excessive protein consumed cannot be used by the body and is transformed into toxic end-products which must be eliminated or else poison the body, we can appreciat the significance of Dr. Hindhede's findings and their immense importance. In his book, "Protein and Nutrition," Dr. Hindhede present the following conclusions, based on his lengthy researches which demonstrated that a low protein diet is best for health, whereas a high protein diet, especially one consisting largely of animal proteins (meat, eggs, etc.) is a definite health menace:

Reasons Why A High Protein Diet is Disease-Producing

1. **Rich protein diet is not only useless but, probably harmful.** I have already said that it would seem to be practically impossible to avoid getting protein enough! Does it not appear to be quite in the order of things that, practically, we must always get enough protein for our needs if we eat as nature dictates?...The first point is that much protein is useless; the second is to discover to what extent and in what way a high intake of protein is harmful.

2. **It is probable that muscular strength declines on a rich protein (Meat) diet.** For evidence I will draw on my own experience. I feel weaker after eating much meat, and physiologists tell us the same story of their test subjects when these are supplied with meat alone. All doctors know how weakening is the effect of a meat diet, such as the diabetic diet and the Banting system.

Protein which cannot be intirely consumed on the body leaves behind it a large proportion of incombustible waste, which is the office of the liver and kidneys to excrete, calling for special exertion on the part of these organs. Now, is this large amount of pprotien be unwanted, unnecessary, it is not a very far step to the assumppion that it must be injurious, because such a considerable amount of energy must be devoted to the katabolism in the cells and to the excretion of its products through the kidneys, energy which might, otherwise be utilized to assist metabolism in the muscles; and in the consequent fatigue we have our explanation.

3. **It is probable that a rich protein diet is the cause of various aliments.** That luxurious habits, especially overindulgence in meat, can give rise to various stomach, kidney and arthritical complaints, is supported by manifold experience. To bring direct proof to bear on it is difficult, for there are so many other factors which may have a contributery effect...It is, however, probable that in these cases, as well as in gout, the trouble arises from poison by the decomposition products of protein. Several of these are poisonous, such as ammonia and nearly related bodies, which form the antecedents of urea...The office of the liver is to render harmless, by conversion into urea, the ammonium compounds which arise from the decomposition of animal protein in the intestines, and suggests that the organ performs the same service in regard to various other waste products of metabolism. It is easy to conceive that the liver is to a certain degree composed of these poisonous products, but that there are limits to the functional ability of the organ to render these poisons harmless, which may possibly explain some of the maladies from which these who indulge largely in meat suffer.

"Appendicitis is, probably, a meat-eating disease. While discussing complaints and their relation to meat-eating, we must not overlook uric acid disorders, such as gout, urinary calculi, etc. That meat contains many purin bodies which are excreted as uric acid is well known; and as meat urine is very acid, the uric acid is not easily dissolved, but is precipitated as a red sediment, to the bottom of the receptacle. Or it may be precipitated beforehand in the pelvis of the kidney, or even in the tissues of the body.

"Potato urine is almost diametrically different from meat urine; it is very slightly acid, being almost alkaline. Uric acid is never precipitated in potato urine, which, on the contrary, is able to dissolve large quantities of added uric acid. The astonishing facility with which potato urine will dissolve uric acid was discovered by the author, quite fortuitously, when conduction extending experiments in nutrition on potatoes. It was discovered for instance, that potato urine, which had been standing for twenty-four hours at body temperature was able to dissolve 3.65 grams of uric acid, while meat urine, on the other hand, could not dissolve its own uric acid, but, to the contrary, precipitated about 1 gram every day. From this it is conceivable that renal gravel could be removed under the dissolving influence of potato urine. Whether a potato diet would be successful in dissolving uric acid which had been precipitated in the tissues of the body I am not yet able to state; but there are indications that it is within the range of probability. Other vegetables and fruits - especially carrots, tomatoes, bananas, etc. - have a similar effect to that of potatoes; while bread has an effect similar to meat.

"This discovery would appear to have settled a long-vexed question concerning diet regulation in cases of kidney stones. Some doctors recommend vegetarian diet, whule others take the opposite course and recommend meat or the usual mixed diet, the latter arguing that certain peoples who are known to subsist on almost exclusively vegetarian diet, such as the Russian peasants and East Indian coolies, are often subject to this complaint. But when we learn that the Russian peasants live chiefly on bread and that the East Indians live mostly on rice, wheat and beans, the explanation is simple enough. Among the poorer classes in Germany, potatoes form the staple food, and kidney gravel is almost unknown. Our observations have shown us that purin-free diet is not a sufficient guarantee against urinary calculus. Bread contains no purin, yet does not serve as any protection against uric acid disorders." (The reason for this is because wheat and most other grains, except millet, corn and wild rice, are acid-forming, and it is the heightened urinary acidity resulting from their use that causes uric acid deposits. Potatoes, on the other hand, being highly alkaline, dissolve and remove the uric acid deposits formed by acid-forming foods as wheat and meat.)

Therapeutic Value of Alkaline Potato Diet

Dr. Hindhede employed alkaline diets consisting of much potatoes and potato water with great success among his patients. One of these patients suffered from gout, his joints being stiff, enlarged and deformed. This condition finally spread over the whole body, the fingers being so cramped that he could not hold anything. Dr. Hindhede put him on a potato diet, consisting chiefly of potatoes and potato water. Though the patient had been sick for fourteen years after four months on the potato diet he was almost well enough to resume work. His fingers, formerly cramped, now were as lithe and supple as a violinist's.

Describing the benefits of Dr. Hindhede's alkaline potato diet, the patient said: "I am sure it was the most potent factor in my recovery. I have experienced a state of health I have not enjoyed for may years."

After reading Dr. Hindhede's book above referred to, "Protein and Nutrition," the writer decided to try his low protein diet using potatoes as his exclusive protein, which he did for six years. During this period he avoided vegetables (because he lived in a city and all vegetables available were sprayed) and ate little else besides potatoes. However, he failed to realize that potatoes, though they grew under the ground and so did not come into direct contact with sprays, nevertheless did contain spray residues, absorbed by the leaf and roots of the potato plant, after these poisons found their way into the soil. For this reason his potato diet was not entirely successful and he was forced to abandon it. (In those days, organically grown potatoes and other foods were not available, since the present organic movement in America was not yet born.)

Remarkable Experiment of Dr. Rose, Who Lived Twelve Years on Potatoes

A German medical man and biochemist, Dr. Rose, lived on potatoes alone for a much longer period, for twelve years, but the potatoes he used he grew himself on his own organic farm, and hence his experiment was unwell, suffering from neurasthenia from which he found no relief. He was then living on a high protein diet. So he secured a farm and planted it entirely in potatoes, on which he lived for a dozen years, using scarcely anything else except occasionally carrots or other vegetables. At the end of twelve years, during which time he lived almost entirely on potatoes, Dr. Rose regained his health, having gotten rid of his neurasthenia. He then wrote a book. "Eisweiss Uberfutterung und Basenuntererhnarung" (Protein Overconsumption and Alkaline Mineral Underconsumption), in which he claimed that the chief cause of most diseases that afflict civilized mankind is excessive intake of protein, leading to acidosis and demineralization, and that the best way to preserve health and increase the body's power of resistance ot disease is to heighten the blood's alkali reserve through a low protein alkaline diet. Let us summarize some of the basic ideas of Dr. Rose's book.

Of all foods, proteins and fats are the greatest acid producers. While starch and sugar forms carbonic acid, a relatively mild acid which is neutralized by the alkali reserve and converted into carbon dioxide, which is eliminated through the lungs, in the case of protein it is different. The metabolic end-products of protein include a number of strong acids - nitric, sulphuric, phosphoric and uric - which cannot be so easily disposed of. They must first be neutralized by combination with alkaline minerals - sodium, potassium, calcium and magnesium - which they rob from the blood, froming neutral salts which must be eliminated through the kidneys. It is clear that consumption of an excess of protein imposes a severe drain on the body's alkali reserve and produces demineralization of the organism. When the formation of these acids exceeds the power of the alkali reserve to neutralize them, a condition of acidosis results, which lays the foundation for a great number of different diseases. These acids are apt to attack any part of the body and predispose to disease in such organs. They may attack and eat away calcium from the teeth, or may withdraw calcium from nervous tissues. producing a state of neurasthenia. This was the condition from which Dr. Rose suffered at the beginning of his experiment, when he lived on a high protein diet. As a medical man, he was taught in college that protein was essential for life and health and that without sufficient protein, the organism will become diseased.

Voit, the German nutritional authority, claimed that the body required 188 grams of protein daily. But in spite of all the protein Dr. Rose ate, his health steadily declined. He got thinner and thinner; and his neurasthenia got worse and worse.

Becoming convinced, as the result of his disappointing experience with a high protein diet, that there was something wrong with orthodox medical belief in the value of such a diet, Dr. Rose gave up his medical practice and decided to regain his lost health by settling on a farm and devoting himself to the growing of organically grown potatoes, on which he lived almost exclusively for a period of 12 years. During this time he ate no meat, no fowl, no eggs and no dairy products, living as a strict vegetarian on a low protein diet of potatoes. At the end of twelve years on potatoes, he enjoyed perfect health and vigor, and then wrote the nutritional treatise referred to.

In his book, Dr. Rose claimed that most of the diseases that afflict humanity came from acid saturation of the blood stream and body issues, whose chief cause is an excessively protein-rich diet. Convinced that the human being is by nature a low protein feeder, Dr. Rose concluded that it is a big mistake to believe that one needs an abundant intake of protein for health and strength. As a matter of fact, excessive protein, by the acid end-products of metabolism which it forms in the blood, really weakens one, since fatigue is a product of acid intoxication more than it is of muscular activity. Dr. Rose claimed that it is a big mistake to consume meat, eggs and other animal foods rich in protein, for then one surely will obtain an excess, which it is more difficult to do when consuming vegetable foods poor in protein, as potatoes. On this latter food, one may obtain all the protein one requires, and enjoy perfect health and normal weight, without suffering any deficiency of protein. This is proof of what a small amount of protein the human body really requires. Since an excess of protein turns the blood acid- and since acid blood predisposes to disease, Dr. Rose concluded that an alkaline low protein diet provides the best security against disease.

Dr. Hindhede's Experimental Subjects Who Lived from 300 Days to Two Years on Potatoes as Their Exclusive Protein

Dr. Rose's twelve year potato diet experiment confirmed Dr. Hindhede's findings which proved that Irish potatoes are capable of serving as an exclusive source of protein in human nutrition, and may be safely used in place of meat and all other proteins, while at the same time supplying sufficient nitrogen. This was demonstrated by the fact that one of Dr. Hindhede's subjects, a young man, lived for 308 days on potatoes and margarine alone, and during this time did heavy work. Describing another case, Dr. Hindhede writes: "My assistant lived 6 months on potatoes, and water, rising part of the year at 3-4 a.m., doing gardening work and working until 10 1'clock at night, once working continuously two days and one night." Dr. Hindhede kept other experimental subjects in his nutrition laboratory in Copenhagen for 300 days on potatoes and oleomargarine alone. All worked hard, and their health greatly improved at the end of the experiment, when they displayed almost undefatiguable energy.

One of Dr. Hindhede's subjects lived for nearly two years on a diet consisting chiefly of potatoes and greens, without fat.

Dr. John Harvey Kellogg describes this experiment as follows, on the basis of a report he received directly from his Danish colleague: "In a letter received by the writer from Professor Hindhede of Copenhagen a couple of years ago, he said that he then had under observation a man who had subsisted for twenty-three months on a diet consisting exclusively of potatoes, bread and greens. No fat of any kind was added to the foods named, and not a particle of other food has been eaten, yet the subject was in perfect health. Professor Hindhede remarked that large quantities of greens are very essential. McCollum, Mendel and others have shown that both cerals and potatoes are deficient in the fat-soluble growth-promoting vitamin, which is supplied abundantly by greens of all sorts."

Influence of Acid-Base Balance on Protein Requirement

Dr. Hindhede's experiments on potato diets were repeated by a number of other eminent nutritionist, including Prof. McCollum at ohns Hopkins University and Rose and Cooper at Columbia University, who confirmed his results. McCollum concluded that potatoes can serve as an exclusive source of protein in the diet over large periods of time, without injury. Thomas experimented with potato diets, and concluded that potaot protein had twice the biological value of wheat protein. The eminent Swedish biochemist, Ragnar Berg, confirmed Hindhede's observation that on an alkaline potaot diet, only 25 grams of protein per day were sufficient, which amount Berg even lowered to 20 grams on a banana diet. But when meat was used as a protein food, he found that over 100 grams per day was necessary. This meant that the protein requirement depended on the acid or alkaline reaction of the diet, a more alkaline diet making for a lower protein requirement and a more acid diet for a higher one. His explanation for this was that the more alkaline the diet and the blood-stream, the less tendency there is for katabolic cellular decomposition to occur, and consequently less wear and tear and loss of body protein, whereas on an acid-forming diet nitrogenous katabolism and loss increases, so that there is greater need for protein intake to replace this loss.

Potatoes as Natural Alkalizers

Dr. Alexander Haig, author of the voluminous medical treatise, "Uric Acid, a Factor in the Causation of Disease", claims that while foods such as meat, fowl, fish, eggs, cheese and wheat, by introducing uric acid into the body, predispose to disease, potatoes, vegetables and fruits, which are alkaline in reaction, protect the body against acid intoxication which causes a great number of illnesses besides rheumatism and the characteristic uric-acid-type disorders.

While he recommends the use of rice in place of wheat, rye and oats, he considers the potato as the best carbohydrate due to its high alkalinity, which makes it a natural alkalizer. He found it to be one of the most effective neutralizers and combatters of uric acid in the system, so that persons who suffer from rheumatism and arthritis, as well as acidosis in general, he believes will greatly benefit by living largely on potatoes, and to use them in place of acid-forming cereals. Dr. Haig writes: "Potatoes, in addition to somewhat less than two per cent of albumen, contribute a considerable quantity of alkali, which is often useful to keep down the acidity of the urine and prevent retention of uric acid by other foods, some of which, such as cereals, have been mentioned as contributing some excess of acids.

"For this reason, eating a moderate quantities of potatoes twice a day may suffice to make a urine which tends to throw out a little red sand from time to time, owing to relatively high acidity, cease to do so, and those who suffer in this way from eating acid fruits should counteract their effects by taking a corresponding quantity of potatoes."

Concerning the value of potatoes as alkalizers, valuable for counteracting acidosis and the many ills that arise from it, and therefore a medicine as well as a food, Dr. Arnold Lorand writes: "When we wish to introduce many alkaline substances into the body, potatoes render good service; large quantities will render the urine alkaline. Moose states that one kilo of potatoes contains almost as much alkaline substances as is present in a liter of Vichy water and he has observed - as is often the case after the use of alkaline waters - that the sugar in the urine of diabetic patients was considerably decreased after potatoes had been eaten, for which reason he recommends a diet exclusively of potatoes for the treatment of diabetes. Especially in northern regions, as in Scandinavia and even more so in Ireland does the potato form a chief part of the daily food. In many sections of northern Hungary, the Slovaks live almost exclusively upon potatoes."

Raw potatoes, according to McCollum, are an excellent antiscorbutic food, due to their high content of vitamin C. Referring to the value of the potato as a preventive of scurvy, Report 38 of the Medical Research Council of Great Britain says: "There is no doubt that in northern climates the potato is of the utmost importance in preventing scurvy during the winter and spring. Epidemics of scurvy have repeatedly followed failure of the potato harvest, e.g., in Norway in 1904 and in Ireland in 1847. The outbreaks of scurvy reported in Glasgow, Manchester and Newcastle in the spring of 1917 are doubtlessly to be attributed to the great scarcity of potatoes at that period." It is also interesting to note that the terrible plagues that swept over Europe during the Middle Ages, taking the lives of millions suddenly ceased following the discovery of America, when the potato was first introduced in the diet, supplying its valuable alkalies, to balance the acid effects of the meat and wheat diet then in common use.

An excellent way to obtain the benefits of the high vitamin C content of the raw potato is to grate it and then prepare as potato patties. By frying in a glass frying pan, and by using virgin sesame seed oil, the usual high temperature of frying, with resulting formation of poisonous acrolein (by decomposition of fat) is avoided, and such potato pancakes are perfectly digestible.

Potatoes are valuable for mental workers because of their high content of phosphorus in combination with potash, both of which are important brain constituents. They also contain lecithin and a lipoidal substance identical with the female sex hormone, which produces typical estrual manifestations in rats.

Constantinidi preformed experiments on potato diets and concluded that "vegetable protein acts no differently in the intestines than animal protein." Carter emphasized the fact that part of the potato nitrogen is in the form of asparagin, which is an anti-putrefactive substance;

and this explains why potatoes are such a baluable antitoxic food, which counteracts constipation and autointoxication. Professor Abderhalden, famous physiological chemist of Halle, says that the potato is a complete nitriment, that is able to support life indefinitely. This was clearly proven in the case of Dr. Rose, referred to before, who gained health steadily during the twelve years that he lived almost exclusively on potatoes.

Good Versus Bad Potatoes: Organically Grown or Sprayed

There are potatoes and potatoes; and Hindhede remarked that the success of his potato experiments depended on whether he secured good or bad ones. In general, practically all potatoes on the general market in this country may be considered as bad potatoes, because they have been grown with chemical fertilizers and sprayed with DDT, or arsenical and copper compounds, as Bordeaux mixture, which is the common spray used against potato beetles. The fact that the tuber is under the ground does not protect it from acquiring poisonous spray residues, since it has been proven that the leaf of the potato plant can absorb poisons applied and transmit them to the tuber. Also after these poisons are washed down by rainfall into the soil, the roots of the plant take them up and transmit them to the tuber. For this reason potatoes on the market contain toxic spray residues which do more harm than the valuable alkalies of the potaot do good. Fortunately there are a few organic farmers in this country growing and shipping organically grown, unsprayed potatoes. These are the only ones fit to eat.

Solanin, a Narcotic Alkaloid in Sprouting Potatoes

But even organically grown potatoes can contain a poison known as solanin, which tends to accumulate when they start to sprout, being present chiefly in the sprouts and around the eyes from which the sprouts arise, as well as in the outer layer of the potato, all of which should be carefully peeled away if sprouting potatoes are used. In some cases, when this was not done, and the entire sprouting potatoe, sprouts and all, was consumed, cases of "potato poisoning" have been known to occur. The potato, like the tomato, egg plant, peppers and tobacco, belongs to the nightshades, a poisonous species. The common idea that peeling the outer layer of the potato removes all or most of its vitamins and minerals is not correct. During the last war, experiments in England have shown that peeled potaotes were quite rich sources of vitamins and minerals which were distributed throughout their substance. It is the fact that potatoes in their jackets are usually baked or steamed, whereas peeled potatoes are generally cooked in water in which their vitamins and minerals dissolve and which are lost when this water is thrown away, that has given rise to this idea. As a matter of fact, while new potatoes with low solanin content, are best baked in their jackets and the whole potato consumed, when potatoes get older and start to sprout, with resulting formation of ever-larger amounts of solanin, a narcotic alkaloid, they are best when first peeled before being prepared. In this way solanin, a natural poison present in the solanes, or nightshade, family is removed, it being present chiefly in the upper layer of the potato.

It is interesting to note that while the Irish potato belongs to the nightshade family, the sweet potato is a member of the morning glory family and is free from any poisonous substance. The same is true of the dasheen (otherwise known as the taro), a member of the caladium, or elephant ear, family.

This tuber has twice the protein content of the potato and has a chestnut-like flavor. It is grown and eaten throughout the tropics. Another tuber which has a white flesh resembling the potato, and which greatly resembles it when cooked, is the tropical yam, a vine-like plant which forms immense tubers, which are free from any toxic or narcotic substance, as present in the Irish potato when it psrouts. Since the solanin of potatoes is to a large extent dissipated under the influence of heat and exposure to air, we can understand why old potatoes should not be baked in their skins, for then, the hardening of the skin during baking prevents their solanin to escape, whereas if they were peeled and then cooked, steamed, baked or fried, their solanin is largely dissipated by exposure to air under high temperature.

Tropical dasheens and yams are now imported to this country and are consumed largely by the Puerto Rican population here. Those who cannot secure organically grown potatoes, or when these are out of season or are too far advanced in sprouting (and therefore high in solanin content, since solanin, while present in greatest amounts in potato sprouts and in the outer layer of the tuber, is also present in smaller amounts throughout its substance, increasing in quantity as the potato gets older), will do well to obtain and use these tropical tubers, which are not likely to be grown with chemical fertilizers or sprays, and are free froj natural poisons, as solanin. They can very well replace potatoes in the diet. (They are for sale by Organic Food Research Associates, 215 Sixth Street, Lorain, Ohio.) Also, from Puerto Rico is imported large baking and cooking bananas known as plantains, the "bread of the tropics," which can also be used in place of potatoes. These may be fried when green or cooked or baked when ripe.

Chapter Nine

SUPER FOODS FROM SUPER SOIL

Preview of New Book To Follow "Super Health Thru Organic Super Foods"

A Review of the Agricultural Discoveries of
Sampson Morgan, Originator of a New Soil Science for the Creation of Organic Super Foods -
a New Method of Soil Regeneration Which Is
Far in Advance of Anything That Now Exists

Healthy Food From Healthy Soil

To have healthy bodies we must consume healthy food, and to have healthy food it must come from healthy soil. This means soil free from toxic substances and harmful bacteria, as introduced into the soil by the use of animal wastes - tankage, blood, manure, etc. Also the soil must be free from chemical fertilizer and spray residues, which tend to accumulate therein.

When plants are grown with an excess of nitrogen by heavy manuring, they tend to undergo a rank growth and acquire a sappy, mineral-deficient structure, which is easy prey to insect pests. They lack keeping quality and flavor. But when they are supplied with an abundance of natural minerals in the form of powdered granite and other rocks, and with trace minerals of marine origin by the use of colloidal phosphate and decomposed seaweed, they develop healthy, mineral-rich, disease - and insect-resistant plants, and the bacteriology of the soil is favorable and free from disease-producing micro-organisms introduced by animal refuse and excrements.

Sick Soil Makes Sick Foods

Sick soil produces sick food and sick food makes sick people. By the use of chemical fertilizers and animal manure, plants are stimulated to a forced growth and lack healthy texture. On this subject, McCrillis writes: "The common use of manure and commercial fertilizers, particularly the nitrate of soda generally employed, produce a rapid growing plant structure and one is sometimes deceived by the apparent luxuriousness of its foliage and other outward characteristics. The process, however, as we shall attempt to show, is largely a forcing process, and not one which will replenish or restore those elements that are essential to healthy plant structure."

In England, Sampson Morgan, founder of the Clean Culture system of soil regeneration along non-chemical and non-animal lines, won first prize at agricultural exhibits by growing vegetables, potatoes and fruits by a new method which involved the non-use of animal manure or chemicals. In place of manure he used vegetable humus, secured from cover crops or leaf mold, and in place of chemicals he used powdered ricks, seaweed and wood ashes. Morgan writes: "Pasteur said that germs cause disease, which they do not. My long continued studies in the dust have convinced me that diseases in soils, plants and men arise from conditions brought about by the introduction of poisons and by imperfect environment....Bacteria do not originate disease.

Their advent is always preceded by the existence of unclean conditions. The eventual existence of filth in the animal and vegetable kingdoms brought the bacteria and micro-organisms of disease, as we know them, upon the scene. Before man and plants discarded the simple life, there was no scope for the presence and activities of the pus cells, and of the bad bacteria, because there were no congenial conditions to entice them and no weak, corrupted internal tissues for them to feed upon.

"Disease is the effort of nature to rid the system of morbid accumulations, and a fast will allow nature to work unhampered in that cleansing process. Then when appetite returns, let the body be fed on clean foods produced by Clean Culture...When man began to eat flesh (a filth food), he began to be diseased. When he began to feed animals on manure-fed grass (a filth food), he introduced pus cells and micro-organisms of disease into the lower animal kingdom. When he began to grow fruits, vegetables and grains by the aid of waste animal matter (a filth food), he infected them with similar destructive agents. As a result of these threefold violations of moral law alone, Nature has plagued his structure with purulent diseases, which have in the majority of cases made life a veritable curse."

Progressive gardeners will agree that fresh manure is bad, and so is fresh tankage, sewage blood and other animal refuse. But many believe that well rotted manure is good, simply because it adds humus to the soil. However, such manure is mineral-deficient, since the minerals of the vegetable material from which it was made have been separated from it in the animal's organism and were given off in the urine. This makes manure a very one-sided and acid-forming product, which acidifies the soil. On the other hand, vegetable humus, as secured from cover crops turned over, supply both humus and minerals to the soil and do not tend to acidify it, as animal manure does. One objection to manure that is seldom mentioned is that since animal secretions contain animal hormones it is possible that these hormones may be taken up by plants and transmitted to humans, having an undesirable effect. Sampson Morgan considers the use of manure as a cause of an acid conditions of the soil, resulting from an excess of nitrogen, which he believes is a cause of disease among plants and animals feeding upon them. (Rodale has lately come to accept this view.) Morgan quotes Professor Potter, who says on this subject: "Susceptibility to disease is influenced by manurial treatment in the vegetable kingdom, and high fertilization with nitrogenous manure lowers the power of the plant or organism to resist infection."

Sampson Morgan writes: "In consequence of my Clean Culture teaching, English medical investigators of not took up the study on the Continent, having found, as others had long previously, that the wounds of soldiers who had been used to a meat dietary do not heal anything like so cleanly or quickly as do the wounds of soldiers who had been used to fruit and vegetable dietary. They also found that the most difficult wounds to heal were those of soldiers who had been used to living upon sewage and manure grown products. I could personally quote scores of cases to prove this, which have come under my personal notice. Awful dangers attend the repulsive use of dead and waste animal matters in the growth of foodstuffs. These highly fed and poisoned soilds are a menace to the health of the people wherever they exist.

"If clean plant foods through a clean soil produce healthy tissues in roots, fruits and grains, and through the consumption of the latter, healthy tissues in the human body, it naturally follows that the use of unclean plant foods through an unclean soil must produce unhealthy tissues in roots, fruits, and grains, and through the consumption of the latter, unhealthy tissue in the human body."

"Though the farmer may turn his sheep into meadows marred with tall over-luxuriant tufts of coarse grass, the sheep avoid and will not eat them, even after the pasture around them has been grazed quite bare. (These tufts result from manure droppings, causing the grass growing there to have a rank growth, but to be unhealthy.) They know instinctively that the short succulent sweet healthy grasses are the most savory and richer in nutrients than the tall coarse bladed stuff, which springs up where the foul carbonate-of-amonia-laden manure has been dumped upon the sward."

The Creation of Organic Super Foods

For the production of mineral-rich, healthy soil that will grow Organic Super Foods, Sampson Morgan recommends the use of rock dust of various kinds, coming from the basic rocks, as granite, gneiss, and porphyry, as well as marl, and for extra dressings, when needed, rock phosphate, limestone and colloidal phosphate, which contains over 20 trace minerals. These dressings of rock powders should be combined with vegetable humus, which supplies humic acid to dissolve the rock minerals and render them more soluble, as well as supports the growth of beneficial soil bacteria and holds moisture in the soil. In addition to rock minerals and render them more soluble, as well as supports the growth of beneficial soil bacteria and holds moisture in the soil. In addition to rock dust and humus, derived from cover crops, Sampson Morgan advises the use of ashes derived from the burning of coarse fibrous vegetation and hardwood, which he called "bonfire ash". Such ashes supply an abundance of readily soluble minerals, until the more slowly soluble rock powders become available.

This is Sampson Morgan's "mineralized humus" system of soil fertilization. He writes: "Granite, a crystalline rock of considerable beauty, is best for enhancing soil fertility and enriching all crops naturally. The disintegrated rock fromed the basis of the soil in the beginning. Soil consists of vegetable and mineral amalgamations, and only with such it is possible to enjoy perfect crops and perfect products. According to my Clean Culture teaching, bonfire ash is one of the mightiest factors in the production of perfectly healthy soils.

"In experiments, by digesting feldspar, hornblende and other minerals in water for a week, from a third to one per cent of the mineral was dissolved out by the water. The ordinary farmer and gardener knows little about the dissolving properties of rain water, or understands that the presence of simple particles of the primary rocks in the cultivated soil are necessary to assure the elaboration of healthy supple tissue in the animal organism."

The author intends to follow this book with a sequel, expounding in detail, the agricultural teachings of Dr. Julius Hensel in Germany and Sampson Morgan in England, two of the greatest agricultural reformers in modern times, who first raised their voice against the use of chemical fertilizers and sprays, developing a system of soil regeneration by which they succeeded in producing vegetables and fruits that were immune to disease and insect pests, and which were larger in size and superior in quanity, flavor and mineral content. In short, by their method they grew Organic Super Foods which will create Super Health in those who feed on them. If interested to secure a copy of this new book write to the publisher.

CPSIA information can be obtained
at www.ICGtesting.com
Printed in the USA
BVHW01*1409100918
527066BV00007B/15/P